MW00649514

The Last Half Hour of the Day

The Last Half Hour of the Day
An Anthology of Stories and Essays
That Have Inspired Physicians

Michael A. LaCombe, MD
Christine Laine, MD, MPH
Editors

ACP Press®
AMERICAN COLLEGE OF PHYSICIANS
PHILADELPHIA

Cover design: Flatiron Industries
Text design and composition: Michael E. Ripca
Printed in the United States of America
Printing/Binding: RR Donnelley

Library of Congress Cataloging-in-Publication Data

The last half hour of the day : stories and essays that have inspired physicians / Michael A. LaCombe, Christine Laine, editors.
p. cm.
Includes bibliographical references and index.
ISBN 978-1-934465-09-7 (alk. paper)
1. Medicine—Literary collections. 2. Physicians—Literary collections. 3. Patients—Literary collections. I. LaCombe, Michael A., 1942- II. Laine, Christine.
PN6071.M38L37 2008
808.8'03561—dc22
2008021295

08 09 10 11 12 / 10 9 8 7 6 5 4 3 2 1

*For Physicians who aspire
to a life-long habit of a half hour's reading
before turning out the light*

…it was at this early period he began his life-long habit of a half-hour's reading in bed before putting out the light. Most medical students, alas, are too engrossed with their work for such literary pursuits, desirable though they may be.

from **The Life of Sir William Osler**

Harvey Cushing

These stories were the libraries of our people. In each story, there was recorded some event of interest or importance, some happening that affected the lives of people. There were calamities, discoveries, achievements, and victories to be kept. The seasons and the years were named for principal events that took place. There was the year of the "moving star" when these bright bodies left their places in the sky and seemed to fall to earth or vanished altogether; the year of the great prairie fire when the buffalo became scarce; and the year that Long Hair (Custer) was killed. But not all our stories were historical. Some taught the virtues — kindness, obedience, thrift, and the rewards of right living. Then there were stories of pure fancy in which I can see no meaning. Maybe they are so old that their meaning has been lost in the countless years, for our people are old. But even so, a people enrich their minds who keep their history on the leaves of memory. Countless leaves in countless books have robbed a people of both history and memory.

Luther Standing Bear, Lakota Indian

Acknowledgements

The following people, from all over the world, sent in their favorite prose for inclusion in this anthology:

Delise Wear John Burnside Rebecca Garden Dan Shapiro Suzanne Poirier William Armstrong Fran Blanc Howard Markel Suzanne Johnson Joseph Fins Richard Thomson Susan Reese Peter Richardson (British Medical Association/Scotland) Elke Galle (Acta Clinica Belgica) Colin Brown Alison Wright (Sheffield, England) Ian Callanan (Dublin) Margaret McMillan (Scotland) Mark Harper (East Sussex, England) Karen Hitchcock (Australia) Richard Kahn Donald Venes Tony Gustafson Geza Simon James Manning Alice Bessman James Wittmer Marjorie Sirridge Chris Brune K. Patrick Ober William Norcross John Yoon Stephen Howlett   Cem Sungur (Ankara) David Sears Lauri Weisberg Sara Newman M.F. Collen Nathan Clifford Eileen Baade Amesh Adalja Dena Rifkin Ellen Kenner Richard Reed Buddha Basnyat (Nepal) Marilyn Maxwell David Nelson Alan Fine John Palmer Martin Donohoe David Elpern Pat Onion Molly Cooke Johanna Shapiro John Bass Audrey Shafer Marcia Childress JoAnn O'Reilly Robert Farnsworth Eric Mukai Jose Gros-Aymerich (Madrid) Marc Straus Richard Berlin Peter Richardson Sarah O'Connor (Scotland) Christine Casey Felicity Reynolds (London) Muhammad Ali Syed Graham Sutton (Leeds, England) Ian Thompson (South Thames, England) Sally Bastiman (Yarm-North, England) Deborah Swiderski John Hillery (Ireland) Christopher Woods (Lancashire, England) Miriam Kennedy (Ireland) Gavin Falk (UK) Ian Holdaway (Auckland) Michael Alms Claudia McClintock Roger Renfrew N. Mumoli (Italy) Dave Lounsbury Nicolas Abourizk Marshall Lichtman Susan Krantz Reuven Sobel Clare Cathcart (England) George Lawrence Allen (Edinburgh) Martin Finkel Gerry Schechter John Hoesing Cathy Cadigan Kevin Kaufhold Joshua Grossman Ehab Kasasbeh Frank Neelon Mary Brandt Arthur Chernoff Kevin Walsh Kevin Martin Dewayne Andrews Stephen Hilty Sachin Goel Ken Hoekstra Faith Fitzgerald John McClenahan Jeremy Baron (London) Patricia Horne (Dublin) Richard Sobel Allan Prochazka Michael Baum Martin Duke Stan Deresinski Howard Holtz Mark Siegel Tom Inui Subramanian Somasundaram (Chennai, India) Glenn Cloquhoun (N.Z.) Daniel Mattox Peter Raich George Allen (Edinburgh) David Mast Shah Abdul Latif (Bangladesh) Herbert Keating David Fisher Jeremy Smith Robin Glassman Daniel Worthley (Australia) Daniel Lewis Edward Harris Warren Kantrowitz Michelle Uhl Charles Perakis Nancy Zurbach

The editors wish to thank as well Tom Hartman, Angela Gabella, Diane McCabe, Robin Glassman, and Margaret Mary LaCombe for their hard work in making this anthology possible. A special thanks goes to David Elpern for his suggestions and advice concerning this collection.

And thanks as well to The American College of Physicians for the vision to publish this volume.

Contents

Section Four: Victories

Section Five: Pure Fancy

Introduction

This anthology is not a reading list for doctors, but rather a book compiled from the suggestions of doctors who do read. As such it differs in kind from any other literary anthology (excepting perhaps its companion poetry anthology *In Whatever Houses We May Visit: Poems That Have Inspired Physicians*).

In response to a call for great literature, those listed in the acknowledgments section of this book sent in the timeless prose that has inspired them. Their suggestions came to us from all over the world and span the centuries from Hippocrates to Lewis Thomas and literary styles from the learned essay of Sir Thomas More to the science fiction of Ursula Le Guin.

Some of these pieces were nominated multiple times: Bauby's autobiography, Selzer's *Brute*, Lewis' *Arrowsmith*, and Carver's *A Small, Good Thing*, are those. Our physician-nominators hold favorite authors: Anton Chekov, Oliver Sacks, Ernest Hemingway, and Lewis Thomas are here—and favorites who are not included in this volume: William Carlos Williams, Ivan Illich and his *Medical Nemesis*, and Tillie Olsen—not here because of editorial constraints and because these writers can be found in other anthologies published for physicians.

There are gems here perhaps unknown to you and difficult to find: the essays of Abigail Zuger, Lorrie Moore's *People Like That Are the Only People Here*, and Carver's achingly poignant and unforgettable *A Small, Good Thing*. It is impossible to pick just one story by Chekhov, but his *A Doctor's Visit* is widely held as one of his finest doctor stories. Susan Mates, a practicing physician herself, is a wonderful writer who should be more widely known. There are several Pulitzer Prize and National Book Award winners here, and seven Nobel Laureates.

The biographies appended at the end of the anthology suggest further reading. Our aim is simple: start with that "last half hour" of Osler, and progress to a lifetime of reading.

Christine Laine, MD, MPH
Michael A. LaCombe, MD
Editors

SECTION 1
Achievements

Life is short
The art long
Opportunity fleeting
Experience perilous
Decision difficult

Hippocrates

Slave Doctors… Free Doctors
(*from* Book IV of Laws)

Plato

And did you ever observe that there are two classes of patients in states, slaves and freemen; and the slave doctors run about and cure the slaves, or wait for them in the dispensaries? Practitioners of this sort never talk to their patients individually, or let them talk about their own individual complaints? The slave doctor prescribes what mere experience suggests, as if he had exact knowledge; and when he has given his orders, like a tyrant, he rushes off with equal assurance to some other servant who is ill; and so he relieves the master of the house of the care of his invalid slaves. But the other doctor, who is a freeman, attends and practises upon freemen; and he carries his enquiries far back, and goes into the nature of the disorder; he enters into discourse with the patient and with his friends, and is at once getting information from the sick man, and also instructing him as far as he is able, and he will not prescribe for him until he has first convinced him; at last, when he has brought the patient more and more under his persuasive influences and set him on the road to health, he attempts to effect a cure. Now which is the better way of proceeding in a physician and in a trainer? Is he the better who accomplishes his ends in a double way, or he who works in one way, and that the ruder and inferior?

from Utopia

Thomas More

Outside their towns there are places located near running water for killing their cattle and for washing away filth, which is done by their slaves. They do not allow their citizens to kill cattle, because they think that pity and good-nature, which are among the best of those affections born in us, are much degraded by butchering animals. They also do not allow anything that is foul or unclean to be brought inside their towns, for fear that the air might be infected by ill-smells which might affect their health. . .

They take more care of their sick than of any others. These are lodged and provided for in public hospitals, of which every town has four. These are built outside their walls and are so large that they might be taken for little towns. By this arrangement, if they ever have a large number of sick persons, they could lodge them conveniently at such a distance that those with infectious diseases may be kept far enough from the rest of the population that there can be no danger of contagion. The hospitals are furnished and stored with all things that are convenient for the ease and recovery of the sick. Those that are put in them are looked after with tender and watchful care, are constantly attended by their skilful physicians, and no one is sent there against their will. As a result, there is hardly anyone in a whole town who, if he should fall ill, would not choose to go to the hospital rather than lie sick at home.

from Letter to Dr. Edward Jenner

Thomas Jefferson

I have received a copy of the evidence at large respecting the discovery of the vaccine inoculation which you have been pleased to send me, and for which I return you my thanks. Having been among the early converts, in this part of the globe, to its efficiency, I took an early part in recommending it to my countrymen. I avail myself of this occasion of rendering you a portion of the tribute of gratitude due to you from the whole human family. Medicine has never before produced any single improvement of such utility. Harvey's discovery of the circulation of the blood was a beautiful addition to our knowledge of the animal economy, but on a review of the practice of medicine before and since that epoch, I do not see any great amelioration which has been derived from that discovery. You have erased from the calendar of human afflictions one of its greatest. Yours is the comfortable reflection that mankind can never forget that you have lived. Future nations will know by history only that the loathsome smallpox has existed and by you has been extirpated.

from The Evolution of Modern Medicine

William Osler

Medicine arose out of the primal sympathy of man with man; out of the desire to help those in sorrow, need and sickness.

> In the primal sympathy
> Which having been must ever be;
> In the soothing thoughts that spring
> Out of human suffering.

The instinct of self-preservation, the longing to relieve a loved one, and above all, the maternal passion—for such it is—gradually softened the hard race of man—*tum genus humanum primum mollescere coepit*. In his marvellous sketch of the evolution of man, nothing illustrates more forcibly the prescience of Lucretius than the picture of the growth of sympathy: "When with cries and gestures they taught with broken words that 'tis right for all men to have pity on the weak." I heard the well-known medical historian, the late Dr. Payne, remark that "the basis of medicine is sympathy and the desire to help others, and whatever is done with this end must be called medicine."

The first lessons came to primitive man by injuries, accidents, bites of beasts and serpents, perhaps for long ages not appreciated by his childlike mind, but, little by little, such experiences crystallized into useful knowledge. The experiments of nature made clear to him the relation of cause and effect, but it is not likely, as Pliny suggests, that he picked up his earliest knowledge from the observation of certain practices in animals, as the natural phlebotomy of the plethoric hippopotamus, or the use of emetics from the dog, or the use of enemata from the ibis. On the other hand, Celsus is probably right in his account of the origin of rational medicine. "Some of the sick on account of their eagerness took food on the first day, some on account of loathing abstained; and the disease in those who refrained was more relieved. Some ate during a fever, some a little before it, others after it had subsided, and those who had waited to the end did best. For the same reason some at the beginning of an illness used a full diet, others a spare, and the former were made worse. Occurring daily, such things impressed careful men, who noted what had best helped the sick, then began to prescribe them. In this way medicine had its rise from the experience of the recovery of some, of the death of others, distinguishing the hurtful from the salutary things" (Book I). The association of ideas was suggestive—the plant eyebright was used for centuries in diseases of the eye because a black speck in the flower suggested the pupil of the eye. The old herbals are full of similar illustrations upon which, indeed, the so-called doctrine of signatures depends. Observation came, and with it an ever widening experience. No society so primitive without some evidence of the existence of a healing art, which grew with its growth, and became part of the fabric of its organization.

M. Myriel Becomes M. Welcome
(*from* Book I of Les Miserables)

Victor Hugo

The episcopal palace was a huge and beautiful house, built of stone at the beginning of the last century by M. Henri Puget, Doctor of Theology of the Faculty of Paris, Abbe of Simore, who had been Bishop of D. in 1712. This palace was a genuine seignorial residence. Everything about it had a grand air,— the apartments of the Bishop, the drawing-rooms, the chambers, the principal courtyard, which was very large, with walks encircling it under arcades in the old Florentine fashion, and gardens planted with magnificent trees. In the dining-room, a long and superb gallery which was situated on the ground-floor and opened on the gardens, M. Henri Puget had entertained in state, on July 29, 1714, My Lords Charles Brulart de Genlis, archbishop; Prince d'Embrun; Antoine de Mesgrigny, the capuchin, Bishop of Grasse; Philippe de Vendome, Grand Prior of France, Abbe of Saint Honore de Lerins; Francois de Berton de Crillon, bishop, Baron de Vence; Cesar de Sabran de Forcalquier, bishop, Seignor of Glandeve; and Jean Soanen, Priest of the Oratory, preacher in ordinary to the king, bishop, Seignor of Senez. The portraits of these seven reverend personages decorated this apartment; and this memorable date, the 29th of July, 1714, was there engraved in letters of gold on a table of white marble.

The hospital was a low and narrow building of a single story, with a small garden.

Three days after his arrival, the Bishop visited the hospital. The visit ended, he had the director requested to be so good as to come to his house.

"Monsieur the director of the hospital," said he to him, "how many sick people have you at the present moment?"

"Twenty-six, Monseigneur."

"That was the number which I counted," said the Bishop.

"The beds," pursued the director, "are very much crowded against each other."

"That is what I observed."

"The halls are nothing but rooms, and it is with difficulty that the air can be changed in them."

"So it seems to me."

"And then, when there is a ray of sun, the garden is very small for the convalescents."

"That was what I said to myself."

"In case of epidemics,—we have had the typhus fever this year; we had the sweating sickness two years ago, and a hundred patients at times,—we know not what to do."

"That is the thought which occurred to me."

"What would you have, Monseigneur?" said the director. "One must resign one's self."

This conversation took place in the gallery dining-room on the ground-floor.

The Bishop remained silent for a moment; then he turned abruptly to the director of the hospital.

"Monsieur," said he, "how many beds do you think this hall alone would hold?"

"Monseigneur's dining-room?" exclaimed the stupefied director.

The Bishop cast a glance round the apartment, and seemed to be taking measures and calculations with his eyes.

"It would hold full twenty beds," said he, as though speaking to himself. Then, raising his voice:

"Hold, Monsieur the director of the hospital, I will tell you something. There is evidently a mistake here. There are thirty-six of you, in five or six small rooms. There are three of us here, and we have room for sixty. There is some mistake, I tell you; you have my house, and I have yours. Give me back my house; you are at home here."

On the following day the thirty-six patients were installed in the Bishop's palace, and the Bishop was settled in the hospital.

Back to Paris
(*from* The Story of San Michele)
Axel Munthe

… Half-way down the Boulevard my friend wanted a bock, so we sat down at a table outside a café.

"Bonsoir, chéri," said the lady at the next table to my friend. "Won't you stand me a bock, I have had no supper." Norstrom told her in an angry voice to leave him alone.

"Bonsoir, Chloe," said I. "How is Flopette?"

"She is doing the back streets, she is no good on the Boulevard till after midnight."

As she spoke Flopette appeared and sat down by the side of her, comrade-in-arms.

"You have been drinking again, Flopette," said I, "do you want to go to the devil altogether?"

"Yes," she answered in a hoarse voice, "it cannot be worse than here."

"You are not very particular about your acquaintances," growled Norstrom, looking horrified at the two prostitutes.

"I have had worse acquaintances than these two," said I. "I am besides their medical advisor. They both have syphilis, absinthe will do the rest, they will end in St. Lazare or in the gutter ere long. At least they do not pretend to be anything but what they are. Do not forget that what they are, they have to thank a man for, and that another man is standing in the street corner opposite to take from them the money we give them. They are not so bad as you think, these prostitutes, they remain women to the last, with all their faults but also with some of their virtues surviving their collapse. Strange to say, they are even capable of falling in love, in the highest significance of the word, and a more pathetic sight you never saw. I have had a prostitute in love with me, she became timid and shy as a young girl, she could even blush under her coating of rouge. Even this loathsome creature at the next table might have been a nice woman had she had a chance. Let me tell you her story.

"Do you remember," said I as we strolled down the Boulevard arm in arm, "do you remember the girls' school in Passy kept by the Soeurs Ste. Thérèse where you took me last year to see a Swedish girl who died of typhoid fever? There was another case in the same school shortly afterwards attended by me, a very beautiful French girl about fifteen. One evening as I was leaving the school I was accosted in the usual way by a woman patrolling the trottoir opposite. As I told her roughly to leave me alone, she implored me in a humble voice to let her say a few words to me. She had been watching me coming out of the school every day for a week, she had not had the courage to speak to me as it was still daylight. She addressed me as Monsieur le Docteur and asked in a trembling voice how was the young girl with typhoid fever, was it dangerous?

" 'I must see her before she dies,'" she sobbed, the tears rolling down her painted cheeks, 'I must see her, I am her mother.' The nuns did not know, the child had been put there when she was three years old, the money was paid through the bank. She herself had never seen the child since then except when watching her from the street corner every Thursday when the girls were taken out for their afternoon walk. I said I was very worried about the child, that I would let her know if she got worse. She did not want to give me her address, she begged me to let her wait for me in the street every evening for news. For a week I found her there trembling with anxiety. I had to tell her the child was getting worse, I knew well it was out of the question to make this wretched prostitute see her dying child, all I could do was promise her to let her know when the end was near, whereupon she consented at last to give me her address. Late the next evening I drove to her address in a street of evil repute, behind the Opéra Comique. The cabman smiled significantly at me and suggested he should come back to fetch me in an hour. I said a quarter of an hour would do. After a rapid scrutiny by the matron of the establishment, I was admitted to the presence of a dozen half-naked ladies in short tunics of red, yellow or green muslin. Would I make my choice? I said my choice was made, I wanted Mademoiselle Flopette. The matron was very sorry, Mademoiselle Flopette had not yet come down, she had of late been very negligent of her duties, she was still dressing in her bedroom. I asked to be taken there at once. It was twenty francs payable in advance and a souvenir à discretion to Flopette if I was satisfied with her, which I was sure to be, she was une fille charmante, prête à tout and very rigolo. Would I like a bottle of champagne taken up to her room?

"Flopette was sitting before her mirror hard at work to cover her face with rouge. She sprang from her chair, snatched a shawl to hide her appalling full undress uniform and stared at me with a face of a clown, with patches of rouge on her cheeks, one eye black with kohl, the other red with tears.

" 'No, she is not dead, but she is very bad. The nun who is on night duty is worn out, I have told her I would bring one of my nurses for tonight. Scrape off that horrible paint from your face, straighten out your hair with oil or vaseline or whatever you like, take off your dreadful muslin gown and put on the nurse's uniform you will find in this parcel. I have just borrowed it from one of my nurses, I think it will do, you are about the same size. I shall come back and fetch you in half-an-hour.' She stared speechless at me as I went downstairs.

" 'Already,' said the matron looking very surprised. I told her I wanted Mademoiselle Flopette to spend the night with me, I was coming back to fetch her. As I drove up before the house half-an-hour later Flopette appeared in the open door in the long cloak of a nurse surrounded by all the ladies in their muslin uniforms of Nothing-at-all.

" 'Aren't you lucky, old girl,' they giggled in chorus, 'to be taken to the Bal Masqué the last night of carnival, you look very chic and quite respectable, I wish your monsieur would take us all!'

" 'Amusez-vous, mes enfants,' smiled the matron, accompanying Flopette to my cab, 'it is fifty francs payable in advance.'

"There was not much nursing to be done. The child was sinking rapidly, she was quite unconscious, it was evident that the end was near. The mother sat the whole night by the bedside staring through her tears at her dying child.

" 'Kiss her good-bye,' said I as the agony set in, 'it is all right, she is quite unconscious.'

"She bent over the child, but suddenly she drew back.

" 'I dare not kiss her,' she sobbed, 'you know I am rotten all over.'

"The next time I saw Flopette she was blind drunk. A week later she threw herself into the Seine. She was dragged out alive, I tried to get her admitted to St. Lazare, but there was no bed available. A month later she drank a bottle of laudanum, she was already half-dead when I came, I have never forgiven myself for pumping the poison out of her stomach. She was clutching in her hand the little shoe of a small child, and in the shoe was a lock of hair. Then she took to absinthe, as reliable a poison as any, though alas, slow to kill. Anyhow she will soon be in the gutter, a safer place to drown herself in than is the Seine."

We stopped before Norstrom's house, Rue Pigalle.

"Good night," said my friend. Thank you for a pleasant evening."

"The same to you," said I.

Last Words

J.P. Featherstone

Some time ago I was called to Richmond to the bedside of an elderly physician. The old doctor was near death and his family had asked whether I would come, would I attend him, was there anything I could do—that sort of thing. I went out of duty more than anything else I guess, that kind of responsibility you have to a colleague.

The man lay in the bedroom of the house where he had lived alone for the past sixty years. Through some minor disappointment—a broken heart or similar tragedy—he had never married. But he was loved nevertheless. Even while I attended him, the constant visits from neighbors and patients were impressive. How could I be of help, I asked the old doctor. His glance and raised eyebrow told me at once that I should know the answer. But if I insisted on staying, he said that I could listen to his story.

And so he began:

"You get to this point, to the end, and all the extraneous stuff of your life just melts away. The picture you are left with all of a sudden gets pretty clear. It's like when you go to the seacoast, you know. You see the boats bobbing in the shallows and the searchlights coming in and out of the fog. There are gulls darting and diving everywhere. And suddenly the fog lifts and there's this leviathan just offshore, right there in front of you for you to see, as honest as the day. Well, that's what this dying does for you. It shows you the leviathans in your life—what was most important to you, what made you who you are. And just as important I suppose, it shows you what has amounted to just so much driftwood through the years.

"I'm lucky I guess. I've had more than my share of leviathans, even more than most doctors I would say. There was that first bright sunny day in medical school on the way to lecture. That's one tremendous leviathan all of us doctors have. And there's the day we all stood on the grass and we were just as green as grass ourselves and we took the Oath together. That's a hell of a leviathan, I'll tell you. And there's your first patient you care for as a full-fledged doctor, and your first life saved, and the first baby you deliver all wriggling and wet and screaming and healthy."

At this point the old doctor's housekeeper entered the bedroom, bustled about, and sent a stare in my direction which said to me in an instant that I was meddling, had no business being there, and should be getting along soon. The house-keeper was either severely kyphotic or a hunchback. I preferred to think of her as a hunchback, possessing magical qualities sometimes bordering on evil and infinite-ly more interesting. At any rate, the old doctor intercepted her look, dismissed it with a wave of his hand, and nodded to me reassuringly.

"You learn so much in this life," the old doctor said, "if you only bother to take the time.

Only after thirty or forty years of experience is a physician really any good at what he does, and by that time he's ready for retirement. That's the great dilemma in medical teaching, how to transmit what the old doctor has learned in those forty years to the young student. It's uncommon these days that medical students and young residents are even put in the hands of experienced clinicians, much less retired practitioners. And it's the uncommon retired practitioner who is any good at teaching anyway. To compound the problem, often the knowledge that he or she has acquired in forty years of experience is often of the ill defined nature: the smell of disease, the nearness of death, the legitimacy of a patient's physical com-plaints, the pathognomonic constellation of signs and symptoms immediately apparent. How can you teach this?"

I began to speak, to give him an answer, but he waved me off, as though there was-n't time, and he had much more to say.

"My God, you'd like to be able to tell them things, like, be an incrementalist. If you take life in small daily bites, in a lifetime you can master French, Shakespeare, and fly-fishing. A day in the doctor's life metaphor for life. You have to learn to plan your day and set priorities, always aware that emergencies, and life, will have quite different plans for you.

"I'd like to be able to tell them that they should choose consciously whether they wish to be a doctor or a businessman. Being a doctor is a calling and requires self-sacrifice, devotion, love and tenderness to your fellow man. If only a kid just starting out could be a doctor without living like one. Keep your overhead low, as the saying goes. Don't become trapped in a lifetime focused on material things. Belief in science, medical knowledge, honing clinical skills, facility with patients, a sensitivity to suffering, a deep love of non-medical literature, a few close friends—these are the important things. The beachfront property, the summer home, the tony private school for your children, the prestigious address, the aca-demic title, membership in exclusive clubs—these are just driftwood, rather silly, if you only stop to think.

"In houses, automobiles and spouses, avoid trophies, I'd tell 'em; you can select a partner who happens to be a trophy, but don't make the selection because of it."

The housekeeper left the room, and the old doctor eased back and became reflective, soft. It was as though he had been filibustering until she left the room.

"Let me tell you what occupies my mind most these days," the old doctor said.

"There is this one particular leviathan bigger than the rest that just wants to occupy my mind.

"It was a long time ago. I had only been in practice for ten or fifteen years maybe. They had a case of diabetic coma over in the hospital in Phippsburg and they called me in to help out. Diabetes was difficult to treat back then. You would administer huge doses of crystalline insulin. All of the fluids you gave were by stomach tube or retention enema, mostly. Oh, sometimes in desperation you'd give a saline solution by clysis, but that never seemed to work. You had only urine tests for sugar and acid to guide you...none of the blood testing you have now. You followed the urines. You looked at the clinical signs. You did your best and prayed. And it seemed that you killed a diabetic just as often as you had one die on you.

"Well this patient, a young woman, was pretty sick. I had to stay with her the better part of a week, walking the thin line between hypoglycemia and ketoacidosis, pouring fluids and alkali into her, injecting the insulin myself. Eventually she responded—youth itself is a great help in treatment, you know. As soon as it was obvious she was going to make it, I turned the case back over to her physician so I could get back to the practice I had left.

"Oh, I'd drive back evenings to see how she was. After office hours I'd like to drop in on her. Her room was always dark. I'd tap at the door and whisper my name and she'd sit right up and ask me to come in. She was a 'good case,' if you know what I mean. You didn't save many diabetics in coma in those days. I guess when you save a life like that you want to bask in it. Well, I'd sit and talk with her for a while and then I'd go out and kid with the nurses and leave.

"After she was discharged I stopped seeing her. I didn't think about her for a while, except maybe to remind myself when I lost a child with meningitis, that I had saved a young woman in diabetic coma."

The hunchback at this point came in with a supper tray, and since there was only one tray, and another more piercing stare, I hastily excused myself.

"Hoyos," said the old doctor. "Come back tomorrow. Get some Hoyo de Monterrey cigars. Excaliburs, if you can find them, 1066's. We'll have a cigar together. I'll supply the Port."

In fact it was several days before I could return to Richmond and to the old doctor's house. The duties of practice, family life and hospital committees had claimed my time at a moment in my life when I was beginning to doubt my own priorities. Nevertheless, he was waiting for me. I had the Hoyos, and he already decanted the Port, a Taylor Fladgate '64. At this point he wasn't about to skimp. The hunchback was in his bedroom, finding things to keep her there, and the old doctor was patently aware of her, yet given to expound again.

"Have you ever noticed how many people envy us?" said the old doctor. "How many people are pretenders to the throne of physician? How many play at being a doctor and yet, consumed by the worst sort of envy, attack us for being so? Have you ever thought about the burden of expectation American society places upon us? I'd like to tell young doctors not to be seduced by it, not to buy into it. Being a good doctor doesn't make you a skillful politician, nor a statesman, nor a gifted teacher, barrister, or philosopher."

I leaned forward to light his cigar— the Hoyos were not easily found, I can tell you—and then sat back in the overstuffed chair next to the sofa he lay upon, and lit my own cigar. Soon the small room was filled with the fragrant clubby haze of tobacco, pungent enough to drive anyone not so inclined from the room, even a hunchback with magical powers.

The old doctor waited until the housekeeper had closed the door behind her, and then his aged face sprang to life.

"The diabetic girl, the one in the coma that I was telling you about the other day," he said, pointing his cigar at me.

"One day she's in my office. She had made an appointment. There she was, sitting in my examining room, just as big as life. Well, I rushed in and we exchanged pleasantries, and she said she had come to thank me for saving her life. Just like that. I said something stupid like it was a thrill for me to manage such a sick patient or something equally sensitive like that. Then I got called out abruptly for a delivery. My nurse gave her another appointment and she was back again the next week.

"'Doctor,' she said just as cool and level-headed as you or I, 'Doctor, do patients ever fall in love with their doctors?'

"Well, I gave her the standard reaction to this, you know, the talk about gratitude and worship and the patient's awe of a doctor's power. I allowed as I could understand any feeling she might have in that regard. I assured her that this was all normal, these feelings she had, and I appreciated it and all that. I think I rambled on quite a bit because she laughed and said,

"'I don't mean to make you nervous, Doctor, but I'm not talking about worship or grateful patients and forgive me for saying this, but I just feel this great love for you.'

"Well, I mean to tell you, I hunted up Freud and ran for cover! I tried to explain to her about father figures. She'd shake her head and say she already had a wonderful father. So I'd bring in transference theory and point out that maybe she had a need for a big brother who could be protective and understanding, and she'd shake her head no again and tell me she didn't need a brother. So I'd say that perhaps I represented qualities that she had been missing in other aspects of her life. She'd smile and nod and agree and I'd see she missed my point entirely. She could have given Susan B. Anthony lessons in persistence!

"Finally I said,

"'Look, you're fifteen years younger than I am. I'm an old man. Look at me! You're a young woman. I mean, just look at me.'

"And that's when she hit me with the ton of bricks. She just looked up at me, or really past me with these innocent brown eyes of hers and said,

"'Don't you know, Doctor?'

"Well, I didn't know. I mean, I didn't know until that very moment. She'd been in a coma after all and then after that, whenever I had visited her in the hospital, it had been at night and her room was dark, so I really didn't know until that very moment that she was blind.

"'I'm sorry,' I said. And she smiled and said that I needn't be sorry, that maybe because she was blind she was more sensitive to people than most and she could pick up things others seemed to miss. She said that she had grown to know me by the sound of my voice and knew just by hearing me talk to her what kind of person I was. She had fallen in love with me, she said, through the sound of my voice."

The old man became quiet, introspective, and visibly upset. I didn't press him. He took a long drag on his cigar, gulped down his port, held his glass to me for more, and said nothing. I was old enough to know better, and so changed the subject.

"Suppose," I said, "Suppose that you were asked to give a lecture to some medical students or young doctors, a sort of Last Lecture. What would you say to them?"

It worked. The old doctor shifted on the sofa, took several quick puffs of his cigar, setting aglow its business end, and literally drowned me in a torrent of seeming non-sequiturs. I only wish now I had tape-recorded it.

"Answer Socrates," he said. "Know yourself. Examine your life. Spend a part of each day in the pure luxury of thinking. Believe in luck. In the role of the cosmic dice, it is pure luck that you were born American and not Bangladeshi, that you hold a blue-chip education, and can move freely in society, rather than having been chained to a system of caste. Be a champion of the downtrodden, the underdog. Don't buy into the specious arguments of high-rollers and certain politicians. The poor and poorly educated do not deserve it. They have not brought it upon themselves.

"And this," he said firmly. He pointed his cigar at me for emphasis. "your family comes first. Not the patient, not your profession, not your career and most certainly not material goods. The secret of a happy, productive physician is the happy, supportive family he or she enjoys. Such support requires an investment in kind. Make no assumptions in this regard. Nor should you postpone love. Tomorrow is never the better time for intimacy." There was a catch in the old man's voice at this last bit of wisdom, and I felt we were close to the diabetic patient once again. I left it alone. There were long minutes of silence. We sat quietly drawing on our cigars, sipping the Port, saying nothing. Then he began again:

"What are hospitals without its plumbers, its maids and laundry personnel, without its maintenance men and janitors, without pharmacists, or aides who empty bedpans, without the compassionate nurses and technicians who believe 'stat' means what it says," said the old doctor. "Without them our university hospitals would grind to a halt. We should recognize them, thank them, bother to know their names. Yet we don't. We should deflect praise rather than searching for it, avoid the limelight. In teaching, it's better to display the brilliance of others, and in caring for patients, I've always tried to give the referring doctor all of the credit— praising him or her to the patient, to the family, and to the referring doctor herself. And along those lines, you should praise publicly, but criticize privately. There is always something good in everyone. Find it, and praise it. And never embarrass a student. Never attempt to show how positively brilliant you are."

The sun was setting behind the expanse of pasture and mountain. The hunchback braved the smoke-filled room with the supper tray. It was time for me to leave, and that moment of what I sensed might be confession was not to come, not today at least.

When I returned in a few days, I discovered I had unwittingly stumbled upon a way to dispel the housekeeper's evil curse. I should have known better. It was her deformity that had thrown me off, but the housekeeper was a woman, after all, and all women love flowers. I had brought a huge bouquet of cut fresh flowers for her, and a box of Hoyos and a bottle of Port for my old friend. "It's a Fonseca," I said, "1976. The clerk said it was the best they had."

"Crack it," said the old doctor. "Life is too short for cheap wine."

"Where were we?" I said.

"I forget," said the old man. He hadn't forgotten, and we both knew it. But he was not about to tell me about the diabetic patient who loved him.

"Your Last Lecture," I advanced.

"Oh, yes," he said, "advice to the young and all that. Well, let's see, here's a passage from my favorite book." He reached over to the low bookshelf, extracted a book, and opened it to where there had been placed a bookmark.

"Here it is," he said, beginning to read.

"'The best thing for being sad.' replied Merlyn, beginning to puff and blow, 'is to learn something. That is the only thing that never fails. You may grow old and trembling in your anatomies, you may lie awake at night listening to the disorder of your veins, you may miss your only love, you may see the world about you devastated by evil lunatics, or know your honor trampled in the sewers of baser minds. There is only one thing for it then—to learn. Learn why the world wags and what wags it. That is the only thing which the mind can never exhaust, never alienate, never be tortured by, never fear or distrust and never dream of regretting. Learning is the thing for you. Look at what a lot of things there are to learn—pure science, the only purity there is. You can learn astronomy in a lifetime, natural history in three, literature in six. And then, after you have exhausted a milliard lifetimes in biology, medicine and theocriticism and geography, history and economics—why, you can start to make a cartwheel out of the appropriate wood, or spend fifty years learning to begin to learn to beat your adversary at fencing. After that you can start again on mathematics, until it is time to learn to plough.'"

"That's beautiful," I said. "Where…?"

"Yes, it is beautiful," said the old doctor, "yes it is. You know, you should never forget what it was like to be a student, how you looked at those senior to you in medical school, what you thought of residents, attendings, seasoned clinicians. We should never forget the power we have over the young people in our profession, a power that can shape lives for good or for evil. And believe me, there is evil in the world.

"Live your life as a Jean Valjean rather than an Edmond Dantès. Seize the opportunity to do The Good Thing. No other profession will give you so many chances. Don't become selfish.

"Selfishness. You know, when I have been racked with guilt, when my soul is as thin and dry as a chip of wood, when I feel worthless and have nothing left to give —when, in short, I have become too selfish, too self-absorbed, I've turned to the cure for these feelings—generosity. I've tried to find someone less fortunate and then was generous to a fault."

I walked into his next diatribe as though he had been lying in wait for me. "You know, only yesterday," I said, " I saw this fabulous movie on television…"

"Instead of one hour before the television set," the old man said, "you could memorize a poem. Think of it. Poetry is the quickest, most efficient way into the thoughts and feelings of a culture or a country. The best words in the best order, as they say. Be careful of that television set," he said, admonishing me, shaking his cigar at me. "Life is what is happening to you while you're getting ready for something else.

"Your favorite poem?" he asked.

" 'Dover Beach' I guess," I said. "Yours?"

"This:
> 'Sometimes things don't go, after all
> from bad to worse. Some years, muscadel
> faces down frost; green thrives; the crops don't fail;
> sometimes a man aims high, and all goes well.
> A people sometimes will step back from war;
> elect an honest man; decide they care
> enough, that they can't leave some stranger poor.
> Some men become what they were born for.
> Sometimes our best efforts do not go
> amiss; sometimes we do as we meant to.
> The sun will sometimes melt a field of sorrow
> that seemed hard frozen: may it happen to you.'"

"Who...?" I asked. But he was ahead of me. The approach of death heightens the senses, as they say.

"The accessible poets, that's what I'd suggest. Dickinson, Frost, Wilbur. And set aside time each day to think. Philosophers do this. You should too. Thinking is not daydreaming. Learn how to think. Your training has taught you how to memorize, and, one hopes, how to learn. But rarely does medical school teach anyone how to think. It requires solitude, thinking does, and you can't find solitude in front of a TV set or at one of your health clubs, or when you're distracted on a busy commute. You need real solitude, and this can teach you focus and concentration, which are vital to thinking."

It was two weeks before I could get back to visit the old doctor again. I have chastened myself since, believe me, over what in my absence I might have missed. Nevertheless, when I went back to see him, the housekeeper greeted me with what vaguely resembled a smile, accepted her flowers, led me hastily to his room, and left us alone. He began to talk about his diabetic patient, as though he had never left off, as though it were the next sentence of his story.

"She stood in my office and just wouldn't leave it alone," said the old doctor. "She said to me, 'I know you, Doctor. I know you very well and I love you with my whole heart. I really do.'

"Lucky for me, I could get called away again and think this thing out. I twisted and turned the whole business around to look at it every way I could. I was her doctor, for God's sake, and I had saved her life after all. Why shouldn't she feel some affection for me? And besides, here I was married to medicine. That's a contract just like any other contract, with rules to follow. You just don't break those rules. You don't allow this kind of thing to happen. You keep your distance. We believed that back then just as you do now. I explained all of this to her and she would just stare off with that wide-eyed innocence of hers and smile and say, 'Why can't I just love you?'

"Well, I didn't give her a return appointment. And she didn't come back to the office again, but something made me drive to her home to see her. I don't know what it was. Or did I? I called those trips house calls at first, but who was I kidding? She was very beautiful, in fact, in a fragile sort of way. I remember being amazed at myself that I hadn't noticed her beauty when I had been treating her disease. Now it seemed that all I could see was her beauty. That, and feel this unwavering love she had for me.

"Okay, I wanted to see her. I had to see her. I was breaking all the rules, cheating on medicine, breaking the Oath. I couldn't help myself. I drove over to see her every chance I could get. I'd take her for walks when there was time...or when her disease would let her.

"I didn't know what had come over me. I would be in my office examining a patient and all of a sudden I'd find myself thinking about her. Or I'd be talking to a family in the hospital and I might be trying to explain to them about this disease their Aunt Martha had and suddenly I'd stop and pause and I'd be off in a day-dream again, imagining myself walking in the woods and kicking the leaves with her. I would get irritated with my secretary if she scheduled patients in at the end of the day because it would mean I'd only get a later start driving over to see her.

"My guilt really bothered me. I don't want you to misunderstand that. It was more than just nice to be with her. It was wonderful to be with her, and I felt almost like I had to be with her, that it was something I lived for, something that was keeping me alive. But I still felt that she was my patient, that I had medicine, that I was married to medicine, that medicine came first, that I had crossed a line I shouldn't have crossed. I would tell her these things. I would tell her that I felt guilty, that this was wrong, that I really shouldn't be doing this, but that I couldn't help myself. She would simply ask me what could possibly be wrong with two people loving each other.

"Her disease didn't just go away. You realize that. She had some pretty bad episodes—imagine what it was like having diabetes before we had any antibiotics. Whenever she was hospitalized, I'd go over and take care of her because there wasn't anyone else qualified to manage her disease and because...she wouldn't have allowed anybody else to take care of her anyway.

"And she became a different kind of patient for me then, I'll tell you! She would teeter on the brink and I would pace and swear...and pray mostly." His voice caught. He swallowed hard, and I could see the tears.

"Isn't it curious that doctors don't believe in God?" he asked me. "But if there is no God, who do you speak to when your patient is doing poorly? And who is it you are whispering to when you are about to stick the subclavian vein, or send home the LP needle, or spark the lifeless heart?

If there is no God, then why is it that patients who are prayed over seem as a group to do better? If there is no God, why is there beauty in the world? If I have learned one thing in forty years of medicine, it is that there is a higher power, and great things unknown to me."

The housekeeper entered with two trays for dinner.

I had arrived.

She left and hastily arrived with a third, joining us for dinner without invitation, without fanfare. She had vased the flowers I had brought her that day and had set them on the sideboard. The fragrance of the paperwhites would not, alas, cut through the cigar smoke. But the housekeeper seemed not to mind. For his part, the old doctor had a full audience now, and although he would refrain from talking about his love, he did not hold back his wisdom.

"How was that meeting you went to?" He gave me no time to answer. "By the way, beware of organizations. Organizations should exist for the common good. But too often they don't. They get caught up in two things. First they try to preserve the monolith above all else; that is, the organization becomes its own first priority. And the second thing, the principal aim of its members becomes self-promotion, when really the members should be working to do The Good Thing."

There it was again, that Good Thing of his. He went on. "To that end, if you find yourself in the unhappy circumstance of belonging to a committee, strive to do The Good Thing, avoid at all costs self-promotion, oppose evil large and small, and in all forms. Speak out, stand for what you believe, fight for the unfortunate, the disenfranchised. In these efforts, be a renegade, a loose cannon, an individual. To become politically adept, a company man, a silent vote for the majority, is to have failed. Oh, you may win titles and position and advancement in the organization, but what have you gained? Remember, there is power in debate and in difference of opinion—in democracy in other words. In 'group-think' there is only death of the soul.

"These organizations that you subscribe to are made up of physicians. And you are a physician so you may have the privilege of caring for others, and of teaching others. For no other reason. Not for some imagined life as a doctor. Not for show, nor ostentation, nor social privilege and position, nor the acquisition of material things. Millions on this earth would give everything they have to trade places with you, for the immense opportunity to do The Good Thing which they now find themselves powerless to do. Don't squander this opportunity.

"Fail one hundred times," he said, nodding to me, "but keep trying. Strive for this on your tombstone:

"'He tried.'"

The housekeeper had left the room abruptly in mid-sentence and was now return-ing with coffee. Since I had consumed three glasses of Port, smoked two cigars, and was heady with the old doctor's wisdom, I could convince myself that the hunchback had added something to my cup, giving my mind this remarkable clar-ity. She left again with the dinner trays and dishes, and as I rose to leave in her wake, the doctor motioned for me to stay. He knew, as I did not, that this would be our last evening together.

"You're wondering what became of her," he said to me. "How it all ended, with me and the diabetic girl. Well, that first winter she was in and out of the hospital all the time, but in spring she was ready for her walks again and I'd drive over to see her every evening. I'd look at my office nurse for some sign of disapproval from her and I knew that all my patients knew something was going on, and I expected the same disapproval from them, but it didn't matter to me.

"We took long walks that spring. She would hold my arm in both of hers and lean on me as we walked. I loved every minute of it. We would talk about the War, about the Brits, about how they were holding out, about how I felt that it was my duty to help them out. I remember the day when I stopped abruptly and turned to her. I held her shoulders in my hands and told her I had to do this thing, I had to go overseas, and I had to do this duty but I would be back, and when I came back I would marry her. If she would have me. I was trying to be all serious and formal and get it right, if you know what I mean. But she just widened her eyes and looked in my direction and threw her head back and laughed and said,

"'Have you? Have you? Of course I will have you!'

"They sent me to a station hospital outside Birmingham. I knew as soon as I got there that I should have married her before I left. War is like dying, you know. It brings everything into focus. It shows you what's important and what's senseless. And what was senseless, I'll tell you, was my worrying about this stupid 'marriage contract' I had with medicine. I mean, lives were ending all around me and the world was falling apart and I wanted nothing else but to be with her. I could only think about her.

"We were very busy at the hospital. I don't think I slept a full night in two years. I managed catnaps whenever I could. They evacuated the wounded over to us— those wounded that survived the trip—and we would patch them up. Believe me, there were plenty of wounded.

"But she never left my mind. I would live for the letters from her, letters she dictat-ed to me, written in her mother's hand.

"We were experimenting with Prontosil, the sulfonamide, you know, treating wound infections with it. The Huns had discovered it a few years before and the Brits had gotten very interested in it. We were using it and having some incredible successes."

He half-turned to me and looked at me and then turned his face and his shoulders to the wall and went on with his story.

"Well, it was ironic that we were using Prontosil, creating all of these miracles with the wounded GI's, and then I get the letter from her mother. It was sepsis. She had died of sepsis.

"Do you know how I felt? I raged at myself! I didn't want to live. I couldn't think. I blamed myself. If I had only married her, if she had been my wife they would have sent me back when she got sick. I could've taken the Prontosil back and saved her life. And she would still be with me. I blamed myself for her death. I should've married her when I had the chance. They'd have sent me back to the States because of a sick wife. But they won't evacuate you for a sick patient.

"I didn't want to go on. All around me the world was fighting for survival and I just wanted to die. I remember walking onto the wards and seeing the GI's lying there, missing a limb or an eye, all wrapped up in their pain, yet managing a smile for me and saying, 'Hi Doc,' and 'Thanks Doc' and...

"I just went on with my life. It wasn't any major decision. I didn't say to myself that well, I'm a doctor and I have Medicine, even though I don't have her. I didn't assume that my decision was made for me, or anything like that. I just put one foot in front of the other and did my job. That's what you do. You just do your job."

I didn't know what to say to the old doctor. After all, he had enough wisdom for three lifetimes. What could I tell him? Oh, I said that I understood, that it was human nature to be cautious, to procrastinate. I talked about all the people in my life whom I had wanted to open up to...be open with...whom I had wanted to understand me. I told him about all of the intended "somedays" in my life when I would relax my guard, would allow myself to feel—those "somedays" that never seem to come. I sympathized with him, about how circumstance has a way of slamming the door on you.

I rose, put a hand on his shoulder, and murmured a goodbye. I was never to see him again. When I returned, with flowers, a few days later, there was a black wreath on the door. I handed the flowers to the housekeeper. She nodded a thanks to me silently, and backed in to the darkened house, closing the door in front of her. I was left alone.

I am now given to long walks, and it is at these times I can be with him again—the old doctor who seemingly broke the rules, and so became human. I walk until the hike exhausts me, and I am flooded by the memory of his words, which are these:

"A physician's professional life is threatened by three enemies: arrogance, greed, and intellectual laziness. Hubris is arrogance dignified. Karl Menninger, the great psychiatrist and doctor of doctors once said that he had successfully treated doctors for every manner of illness—substance abuse, marital discord, depression—but had never been able to cure a physician of greed.

"Never ignore a sign or symptom you can't explain.

"Honesty is fitting words to the actions. Integrity is fitting actions to the words. Our actions define us; not principles, not goals, not titles nor academic rank.

"Approach each patient with this thought in mind: I will learn one single new thing from this person.

"Travel. You must visit other universities, other medical centers, other countries, if only to gain an idea of medicine's differences and its commonalties. To remain provincial is to become both arrogant and ignorant.

"Study medical history. Find your place in it.

"Cultivate your teachers well. Have them teach you how to learn, not spoon-feed you. Cultivate your consultants as well. Do not abuse them. Send them the baffling case you cannot diagnose by your own wit. Do not, out of sheer laziness or crunch of time, send headaches to the neurologist, chest pain to the cardiologist, or arthritis to the rheumatologist. Finally, cultivate your students. Do not try to make them into your own image for purposes of self-affirmation. You will harm them in doing so. Bother to find out what they need and want to do, and what they are capable of. For students, as for children, quality time is all that is required.

"Just as you cannot cure all disease, you cannot be a doctor to all patients. For your own piece of mind and for the well-being of patients, you must learn to say "no", and "I am sorry I cannot help you" and "I think it is time you saw someone else". These may be the most difficult things for a physician to say, reared as she is in a world of omnipotence and endless possibilities.

"Communicate. Imagination is the great demon of marriages, partnerships, universities.

"Be on time. Never punish the prompt.

"If you cannot make a diagnosis, make a decision.' A corollary to this is that most things get better by morning. And its antithesis is this: that if you cannot do something, order a test.

"When in doubt, return to first principles. Take a history. Examine the patient. Talk to the family. Ask the nurse.

"Simplify your life. Thoreau was right. Material possessions will possess you. Acquire an object for its utility, not for its appearance. Measure your worth not in things, but in knowledge and in kindness to others.

"Remember this: 'All that is required for evil to triumph is for good people to do nothing.'

"There is too much to know. Learn what you love and leave the rest to others. Libraries are repositories of knowledge. You are not and cannot be, so don't try to be.

For God's sake, stop pitying yourself. The Great Plague of our ancestors killed doctors. Ours does not. Likely you will never be exposed to the Ebola virus. You are not at the mercy of a despotic king. You are neither bound by class, nor diminished by poverty. You have great science as a tool, not leeches. The excellence of your pharmacy dwarfs arsenic, antimony, belladonna. Your citizenry in the richest, most advanced country in the history of the world is no more than sheer good fortune. You do not live in Uganda. You enjoy more than an ox for transportation. Your children will almost certainly reach adulthood.

"Do not waste your time. Be sensitive to anything that threatens to waste your time, and avoid it. Friends are not a waste of time. Nor is family. Nor is thinking. Nor are matters of the spirit and soul.

"Let your children, your spouse, your colleagues, partners and students, overhear you praising them.

"Stay in shape. This means more than mere diet and exercise. You need a diet of poetry and literature, and stiff exercise in thinking and spiritual contemplation.

"Being a doctor requires quick reflexes. The occasion is instant. Hone your reflexes by a regular habit of exposure to patients, talking to them, touching them, taking a history and doing a physical examination.

"Learn how to listen. You cannot understand another, nor take a meaningful history, by talking.

"Avoid arrogance. In the great panoply of human history, what have you to be proud of?

"We exist for each other. Teach others, care for them. Generosity, that's the key.

"When you begin to become overly proud, when you begin to strut and show, ask yourself this: With the tools available at the time, would you have been capable of the observation and description of Hippocrates, the precision and analysis of Sydenham, the auscultatory skill of Laennec?

"Whatever did we do without evidence-based medicine? How did the giants of medicine practice, after all? Well, I believe this: they were inclined to think."

These were great lessons for me. On my long walks, recalling those hours with him, I can begin to believe myself capable of owning a mere portion of them. Even if only a very small portion.

But if there is one certain lesson I have learned from my days spent with the old doctor and his housekeeper, it is this: Commonly, when I return home to my wife, who is a trophy, but whom I did not marry because she is a trophy, I bring her flowers. A lot of them.

from Arrowsmith

Sinclair Lewis

"To be a scientist—it is not just a different job, so that a man should choose between being a scientist and being an explorer or a bond-salesman or a physician or a king or a farmer. It is a tangle of very obscure emotions, like mysticism, or wanting to write poetry; it makes its victim all different from the good normal man. The normal man, he does not care much what he does except that he should eat and sleep and make love. But the scientist is intensely religious—he is so religious that he will not accept quarter-truths, because they are an insult to his faith.

"He wants that everything should be subject to inexorable laws. He is equal opposed to the capitalists who t'ink their silly money-grabbing is a system, and to liberals who t'ink man is not a fighting animal; he takes both the American booster and the European aristocrat, and he ignores all their blithering. Ignores it! All of it! He hates the preachers who talk their fables, but he iss not too kindly to the anthropologists and historians who can only make guesses, yet they have the nerf to call themselves scientists! Oh, yes, he is a man that all nice good-natured people should naturally hate!

"He speaks no meaner of the ridiculous faith-healers and chiropractors than he does of the doctors that want to snatch our science before it is tested and rush around hoping they heal people, and spoiling all the clues with their footsteps; and worse than the men like hogs, worse than the imbeciles who have not even heard of science, he hates pseudo-scientists, guess-scientists—like these psycho-analysts; and worse than those comic dream-scientists he hates the men that are allowed in a clean kingdom like biology but know only one text-book and how to lecture to nincompoops all so popular! He is the only real revolutionary, the authentic scientist, because he alone knows how liddle he knows.

"He must be heartless. He lives in a cold, clear light. Yes dis is a funny t'ing: really, in private, he is not cold nor heartless—so much less cold than the Professional Optimists. The world has always been ruled by the Philanthropists: by the doctors that want to use therapeutic methods they do not understand, by the soldiers that want something to defend their country against, by the preachers that yearn to make everybody listen to them, by the kind manufacturers that love their workers, by the eloquent statesmen and soft-hearted authors—and see once what a fine mess of hell they haf made of the world! Maybe now it is time for the scientist, who works and searches and never goes around howling how he loves everybody!

"But once again always remember that not all the men who work at science are scientists. So few! The rest—secretaries, press-agents, camp-followers! To be a scientist is like being a Goethe: it is born in you. Sometimes I t'ink you have a liddle of it born in you. If you haf, there is only one t'ing—no, there is two t'ings you must do: work twice as hard as you can, and keep people from using you. I will try to protect you from Success. It is all I can do. So.... I should wish, Martin, that you will be very happy here. May Koch bless you!

Towards the Splendid City

Pablo Neruda

My speech is going to be a long journey, a trip that I have taken through regions that are distant and antipodean, but not for that reason any less similar to the landscape and the solitude in Scandinavia. I refer to the way in which my country stretches down to the extreme South. So remote are we Chileans that our boundaries almost touch the South Pole, recalling the geography of Sweden, whose head reaches the snowy northern region of this planet.

Down there on those vast expanses in my native country, where I was taken by events which have already fallen into oblivion, one has to cross, and I was compelled to cross, the Andes to find the frontier of my country with Argentina. Great forests make these inaccessible areas like a tunnel through which our journey was secret and forbidden, with only the faintest signs to show us the way. There were no tracks and no paths, and I and my four companions, riding on horseback, pressed forward on our tortuous way, avoiding the obstacles set by huge trees, impassable rivers, immense cliffs and desolate expanses of snow, blindly seeking the quarter in which my own liberty lay. Those who were with me knew how to make their way forward between the dense leaves of the forest, but to feel safer they marked their route by slashing with their machetes here and there in the bark of the great trees, leaving tracks which they would follow back when they had left me alone with my destiny.

Each of us made his way forward filled with this limitless solitude, with the green and white silence of trees and huge trailing plants and layers of soil laid down over centuries, among half-fallen tree trunks which suddenly appeared as fresh obstacles to bar our progress. We were in a dazzling and secret world of nature which at the same time was a growing menace of cold, snow and persecution. Everything became one: the solitude, the danger, the silence, and the urgency of my mission.

Sometimes we followed a very faint trail, perhaps left by smugglers or ordinary criminals in flight, and we did not know whether many of them had perished, surprised by the icy hands of winter, by the fearful snowstorms which suddenly rage in the Andes and engulf the traveller, burying him under a whiteness seven storeys high.

On either side of the trail I could observe in the wild desolation something which betrayed human activity. There were piled up branches which had lasted out many winters, offerings made by hundreds who had journeyed there, crude burial mounds in memory of the fallen, so that the passer should think of those who had not been able to struggle on but had remained there under the snow for ever. My comrades, too, hacked off with their machetes branches which brushed our heads and bent down over us from the colossal trees, from oaks whose last leaves were scattering before the winter storms. And I too left a tribute at every mound, a visiting card of wood, a branch from the forest to deck one or other of the graves of these unknown travellers.

We had to cross a river. Up on the Andean summits there run small streams which cast themselves down with dizzy and insane force, forming waterfalls that stir up earth and stones with the violence they bring with them from the heights. But this time we found calm water, a wide mirrorlike expanse which could be forded. The horses splashed in, lost their foothold and began to swim towards the other bank. Soon my horse was almost completely covered by the water, I began to plunge up and down without support, my feet fighting desperately while the horse struggled to keep its head above water. Then we got across. And hardly we reached the further bank when the seasoned countryfolk with me asked me with scarce-concealed smiles:

"Were you frightened?"

"Very. I thought my last hour had come", I said.

"We were behind you with our lassoes in our hands", they answered.

"Just there", added one of them, "my father fell and was swept away by the current. That didn't happen to you."

We continued till we came to a natural tunnel which perhaps had been bored through the imposing rocks by some mighty vanished river or created by some tremor of the earth when these heights had been formed, a channel that we entered where it had been carved out in the rock in granite. After only a few steps our horses began to slip when they sought for a foothold in the uneven surfaces of the stone and their legs were bent, sparks flying from beneath their iron shoes—several times I expected to find myself thrown off and lying there on the rock. My horse was bleeding from its muzzle and from its legs, but we persevered and continued on the long and difficult but magnificent path.

There was something awaiting us in the midst of this wild primeval forest. Suddenly, as if in a strange vision, we came to a beautiful little meadow huddled among the rocks: clear water, green grass, wild flowers, the purling of brooks and the blue heaven above, a generous stream of light unimpeded by leaves.

There we stopped as if within a magic circle, as if guests within some hallowed place, and the ceremony I now took part in had still more the air of something sacred. The cowherds dismounted from their horses. In the midst of the space, set up as if in a rite, was the skull of an ox. In silence the men approached it one after the other and put coins and food in the eyesockets of the skull. I joined them in this sacrifice intended for stray travellers, all kinds of refugees who would find bread and succour in the dead ox's eye sockets.

But the unforgettable ceremony did not end there. My country friends took off their hats and began a strange dance, hopping on one foot around the abandoned skull, moving in the ring of footprints left behind by the many others who had passed there before them. Dimly I understood, there by the side of my inscrutable companions, that there was a kind of link between unknown people, a care, an appeal and an answer even in the most distant and isolated solitude of this world.

Further on, just before we reached the frontier which was to divide me from my native land for many years, we came at night to the last pass between the mountains. Suddenly we saw the glow of a fire as a sure sign of a human presence, and when we came nearer we found some half-ruined buildings, poor hovels which seemed to have been abandoned. We went into one of them and saw the glow of fire from tree trunks burning in the middle of the floor, carcasses of huge trees, which burnt there day and night and from which came smoke that made its way up through the cracks in the roof and rose up like a deep-blue veil in the midst of the darkness. We saw mountains of stacked cheeses, which are made by the people in these high regions. Near the fire lay a number of men grouped like sacks. In the silence we could distinguish the notes of a guitar and words in a song which was born of the embers and the darkness, and which carried with it the first human voice we had encountered during our journey. It was a song of love and distance, a cry of love and longing for the distant spring, from the towns we were coming away from, for life in its limitless extent. These men did not know who we were, they knew nothing about our flight, they had never heard either my name or my poetry; or perhaps they did, perhaps they knew us? What actually happened was that at this fire we sang and we ate, and then in the darkness we went into some primitive rooms. Through them flowed a warm stream, volcanic water in which we bathed, warmth which welled out from the mountain chain and received us in its bosom.

Happily we splashed about, dug ourselves out, as it were, liberated ourselves from the weight of the long journey on horseback. We felt refreshed, reborn, baptised, when in the dawn we started on the journey of a few miles which was to eclipse me from my native land. We rode away on our horses singing, filled with a new air, with a force that cast us out on to the world's broad highway which awaited me. This I remember well, that when we sought to give the mountain dwellers a few coins in gratitude for their songs, for the food, for the warm water, for giving us lodging and beds, I would rather say for the unexpected heavenly refuge that had met us on our journey, our offering was rejected out of hand. They had been at our service, nothing more. In this taciturn "nothing" there were hidden things that were understood, perhaps a recognition, perhaps the same kind of dreams.

Ladies and Gentlemen,

I did not learn from books any recipe for writing a poem, and I, in my turn, will avoid giving any advice on mode or style which might give the new poets even a drop of supposed insight. When I am recounting in this speech something about past events, when reliving on this occasion a never-forgotten occurrence, in this place which is so different from what that was, it is because in the course of my life I have always found somewhere the necessary support, the formula which had been waiting for me not in order to be petrified in my words but in order to explain me to myself.

During this long journey I found the necessary components for the making of the poem. There I received contributions from the earth and from the soul. And I believe that poetry is an action, ephemeral or solemn, in which there enter as equal partners solitude and solidarity, emotion and action, the nearness to oneself, the nearness to mankind and to the secret manifestations of nature. And no less strongly I think that all this is sustained—man and his shadow, man and his conduct, man and his poetry—by an ever-wider sense of community, by an effort which will for ever bring together the reality and the dreams in us because it is precisely in this way that poetry unites and mingles them. And therefore I say that I do not know, after so many years, whether the lessons I learned when I crossed a daunting river, when I danced around the skull of an ox, when I bathed my body in the cleansing water from the topmost heights—I do not know whether these lessons welled forth from me in order to be imparted to many others or whether it was all a message which was sent to me by others as a demand or an accusation. I do not know whether I experienced this or created it, I do not know whether it was truth or poetry, something passing or permanent, the poems I experienced in this hour, the experiences which I later put into verse.

From all this, my friends, there arises an insight which the poet must learn through other people. There is no insurmountable solitude. All paths lead to the same goal: to convey to others what we are. And we must pass through solitude and difficulty, isolation and silence in order to reach forth to the enchanted place where we can dance our clumsy dance and sing our sorrowful song—but in this dance or in this song there are fulfilled the most ancient rites of our conscience in the awareness of being human and of believing in a common destiny.

The truth is that even if some or many consider me to be a sectarian, barred from taking a place at the common table of friendship and responsibility, I do not wish to defend myself, for I believe that neither accusation nor defence is among the tasks of the poet. When all is said, there is no individual poet who administers poetry, and if a poet sets himself up to accuse his fellows or if some other poet wastes his life in defending himself against reasonable or unreasonable charges, it is my conviction that only vanity can so mislead us. I consider the enemies of poetry to be found not among those who practise poetry or guard it but in mere lack of agreement in the poet. For this reason no poet has any considerable enemy other than his own incapacity to make himself understood by the most forgotten and exploited of his contemporaries, and this applies to all epochs and in all countries.

The poet is not a "little god". No, he is not a "little god". He is not picked out by a mystical destiny in preference to those who follow other crafts and professions. I have often maintained that the best poet is he who prepares our daily bread: the nearest baker who does not imagine himself to be a god. He does his majestic and unpretentious work of kneading the dough, consigning it to the oven, baking it in golden colours and handing us our daily bread as a duty of fellowship. And, if the poet succeeds in achieving this simple consciousness, this too will be transformed into an element in an immense activity, in a simple or complicated structure which constitutes the building of a community, the changing of the conditions which surround mankind, the handing over of mankind's products: bread, truth, wine, dreams. If the poet joins this never-completed struggle to extend to the hands of each and all his part of his undertaking, his effort and his tenderness to the daily work of all people, then the poet must take part, the poet will take part, in the sweat, in the bread, in the wine, in the whole dream of humanity. Only in this indispensable way of being ordinary people shall we give back to poetry the mighty breadth which has been pared away from it little by little in every epoch, just as we ourselves have been whittled down in every epoch.

The mistakes which led me to a relative truth and the truths which repeatedly led me back to the mistakes did not allow me—and I never made any claims to it—to find my way to lead, to learn what is called the creative process, to reach the heights of literature that are so difficult of access. But one thing I realized—that it is we ourselves who call forth the spirits through our own myth-making. From the matter we use, or wish to use, there arise later on obstacles to our own development and the future development. We are led infallibly to reality and realism, that is to say to become indirectly conscious of everything that surrounds us and of the ways of change, and then we see, when it seems to be late, that we have erected such an exaggerated barrier that we are killing what is alive instead of helping life to develop and blossom. We force upon ourselves a realism which later proves to be more burdensome than the bricks of the building, without having erected the building which we had regarded as an indispensable part of our task. And, in the contrary case, if we succeed in creating the fetish of the incomprehensible (or the fetish of that which is comprehensible only to a few), the fetish of the exclusive and the secret, if we exclude reality and its realistic degenerations, then we find ourselves suddenly surrounded by an impossible country, a quagmire of leaves, of mud, of cloud, where our feet sink in and we are stifled by the impossibility of communicating.

As far as we in particular are concerned, we writers within the tremendously far-flung American region, we listen unceasingly to the call to fill this mighty void with beings of flesh and blood. We are conscious of our duty as fulfillers—at the same time we are faced with the unavoidable task of critical communication within a world which is empty and is not less full of injustices, punishments and sufferings because it is empty—and we feel also the responsibility for reawakening the old dreams which sleep in statues of stone in the ruined ancient monuments, in the wide-stretching silence in planetary plains, in dense primeval forests, in rivers which roar like thunder. We must fill with words the most distant places in a dumb continent and we are intoxicated by this task of making fables and giving names. This is perhaps what is decisive in my own humble case, and if so my exaggerations or my abundance or my rhetoric would not be anything other than the simplest of events within the daily work of an American. Each and every one of my verses has chosen to take its place as a tangible object, each and every one of my poems has claimed to be a useful working instrument, each and every one of my songs has endeavoured to serve as a sign in space for a meeting between paths which cross one another, or as a piece of stone or wood on which someone, some others, those who follow after, will be able to carve the new signs.

By extending to these extreme consequences the poet's duty, in truth or in error, I determined that my posture within the community and before life should be that of in a humble way taking sides. I decided this when I saw so many honourable misfortunes, lone victories, splendid defeats. In the midst of the arena of America's struggles I saw that my human task was none other than to join the extensive forces of the organized masses of the people, to join with life and soul with suffering and hope, because it is only from this great popular stream that the necessary changes can arise for the authors and for the nations. And even if my attitude gave and still gives rise to bitter or friendly objections, the truth is that I can find no other way for an author in our far-flung and cruel countries, if we want the darkness to blossom, if we are concerned that the millions of people who have learnt neither to read us nor to read at all, who still cannot write or write to us, are to feel at home in the area of dignity without which it is impossible for them to be complete human beings.

We have inherited this damaged life of peoples dragging behind them the burden of the condemnation of centuries, the most paradisaical of peoples, the purest, those who with stones and metals made marvellous towers, jewels of dazzling brilliance—peoples who were suddenly despoiled and silenced in the fearful epochs of colonialism which still linger on.

Our original guiding stars are struggle and hope. But there is no such thing as a lone struggle, no such thing as a lone hope. In every human being are combined the most distant epochs, passivity, mistakes, sufferings, the pressing urgencies of our own time, the pace of history. But what would have become of me if, for example, I had contributed in some way to the maintenance of the feudal past of the great American continent? How should I then have been able to raise my brow, illuminated by the honour which Sweden has conferred on me, if I had not been able to feel some pride in having taken part, even to a small extent, in the change which has now come over my country? It is necessary to look at the map of America, to place oneself before its splendid multiplicity, before the cosmic generosity of the wide places which surround us, in order to understand why many writers refuse to share the dishonour and plundering of the past, of all that which dark gods have taken away from the American peoples.

I chose the difficult way of divided responsibility and, rather than to repeat the worship of the individual as the sun and centre of the system, I have preferred to offer my services in all modesty to an honourable army which may from time to time commit mistakes but which moves forward unceasingly and struggles every day against the anachronism of the refractory and the impatience of the opinionated. For I believe that my duties as a poet involve friendship not only with the rose and with symmetry, with exalted love and endless longing, but also with unrelenting human occupations which I have incorporated into my poetry.

It is today exactly one hundred years since an unhappy and brilliant poet, the most awesome of all despairing souls, wrote down this prophecy: "A l'aurore, armés d'une ardente patience, nous entrerons aux splendides Villes." "In the dawn, armed with a burning patience, we shall enter the splendid Cities."

I believe in this prophecy of Rimbaud, the Visionary. I come from a dark region, from a land separated from all others by the steep contours of its geography. I was the most forlorn of poets and my poetry was provincial, oppressed and rainy. But always I had put my trust in man. I never lost hope. It is perhaps because of this that I have reached as far as I now have with my poetry and also with my banner.

Lastly, I wish to say to the people of good will, to the workers, to the poets, that the whole future has been expressed in this line by Rimbaud: only with a burning patience can we conquer the splendid City which will give light, justice and dignity to all mankind.

In this way the song will not have been sung in vain.

Discoveries

Make it a rule never to be angry at anything a sick man says or does to you.

Sickness often adds to the natural irritability of the temper. We are, therefore, to bear the reproaches of our patients with meekness and silence. It is folly to resent injuries at any time, but it is cowardice to resent an injury from a sick man, since, from his weakness and dependence upon us, he is unable to contend with us upon equal terms.

Benjamin Rush, MD (1809)

Brute

Richard Selzer

You must never again set your anger upon a patient. You were tired, you said, and therefore it happened. Now that you have excused yourself, there is no need for me to do it for you.

Imagine that you yourself go to a doctor because you have chest pain. You are worried that there is something the matter with your heart. Chest pain is your Chief Complaint. It happens that your doctor has been awake all night with a patient who has been bleeding from a peptic ulcer of his stomach. He is tired. That is your doctor's Chief Complaint. I have chest pain, you tell him. I am tired, he says.

Still I confess to some sympathy for you. I know what tired is.

Listen: It is twenty-five years ago in the Emergency Room. It is two o'clock in the morning. There has been a day and night of stabbings, heart attacks and automobile accidents. A commotion at the door: A huge black man is escorted by four policemen into the Emergency Room. He is handcuffed. At the door, the man rears as though to shake off the men who cling to his arms and press him from the rear. Across the full length of his forehead is a laceration. It is deep to the bone. I know it even without probing its depths. The split in his black flesh is like the white wound of an ax in the trunk of a tree. Again and again he throws his head and shoulders forward, then back, rearing, roaring. The policemen ride him like parasites. Had he horns he would gore them. Blind and trussed, the man shakes them about, rattles them. But if one of them loses his grip, the others are still fixed and sucking. The man is hugely drunk—toxic, fuming, murderous—a great mythic beast broken loose in the city, surprised in his night raid by a phalanx of legionnaires armed with clubs and revolvers.

I do not know the blow that struck him on the brow. Or was there any blow? Here is a brow that might have burst on its own, spilling out its excess of rage, bleeding itself toward ease. Perhaps it was done by a jealous lover, a woman, or a man who will not pay him the ten dollars he won on a bet, or still another who has hurled the one insult that he cannot bear to hear. Perhaps it was done by the police themselves. From the distance of many years and from the safety of my little study, I choose to see it thus:

The helmeted corps rounds the street corner. A shout. "There he is!" And they clatter toward him. He stands there for a moment, lurching. Something upon which he had been feeding falls from his open mouth. He turns to face the policemen. For him it is not a new challenge. He is scarred as a Zulu from his many battles. Almost from habit he ascends to the combat. One or more of them falls under his flailing arms until—there is the swing of a truncheon, a sound as though a melon has been dropped from a great height. The white wedge appears upon the sweating brow of the black man, a waving fall of blood pours across his eyes and cheeks.

The man is blinded by it; he is stunned. Still he reaches forth to make contact with the enemy, to do one more piece of damage. More blows to the back, the chest and again to the face. Bloody spume flies from his head as though lifted by a great wind. The police are spattered with it. They stare at each other with an abstract horror and disgust. One last blow, and, blind as Samson, the black man undulates, rolling in a splayfooted circle. But he does not go down. The police are upon him then, pinning him, cuffing his wrists, kneeing him toward the van. Through the back window of the wagon—a netted panther.

In the Emergency Room he is led to the treatment area and to me. There is a vast dignity about him. He keeps his own counsel. What is he thinking? I wonder. The police urge him up on the table. They put him down. They restrain his arms with straps. I examine the wound, and my heart sinks. It is twelve centimeters long, irregular, jagged and, as I knew, to the skull. It will take at least two hours.

I am tired. Also to the bone. But something else ... Oh, let me not deny it. I am ravished by the sight of him, the raw, untreated flesh, his very wildness which suggests less a human than a great and beautiful animal. As though by the addition of the wound, his body is more than it was, more of a body. I begin to cleanse and debride the wound. At my touch, he stirs and groans. "Lie still," I tell him. But now he rolls his head from side to side so that I cannot work. Again and again he lifts his pelvis from the table, strains against his bonds, then falls heavily. He roars something, not quite language. "Hold still," I say. "I cannot stitch your forehead unless you hold still."

Perhaps it is the petulance in my voice that makes him resume his struggle against all odds to be free. Perhaps he understands that it is only a cold, thin official voice such as mine, and not the billy clubs of half-a-dozen cops that can rob him of his dignity. And so he strains and screams. But why can he not sense that I am tired? He spits and curses and rolls his head to escape from my fingers. It is quarter to three in the morning. I have not yet begun to stitch. I lean close to him; his steam fills my nostrils. "Hold still," I say.

"You fuckin' hold still," he says to me in a clear, fierce voice.

Suddenly, I am in the fury with him. Somehow he has managed to capture me, to pull me inside his cage. Now we are two brutes hissing and batting at each other. But I do not fight fairly.

I go to the cupboard and get from it two packets of heavy, braided silk suture and a large curved needle. I pass one of the heavy silk sutures through the eye of the needle. I take the needle in the jaws of a needle holder, and I pass the needle through the center of his right earlobe. Then I pass the needle through the mattress of the stretcher. And I tie the thread tightly so that his head is pulled to the right. I do exactly the same to his left earlobe, and again I tie the thread tightly so that his head is facing directly upward.

"I have sewn your ears to the stretcher," I say. "Move, and you'll rip 'em off." And leaning close I say in a whisper, "Now you fuckin' hold still."

I do more. I wipe the gelatinous clots from his eyes so that he can see. And I lean over him from the head of the table, so that my face is directly above his, upside down. And I grin. It is the cruelest grin of my life. Torturers must grin like that, beheaders and operators of racks.

But now he does hold still. Surely it is not just fear of tearing his earlobes. He is too deep into his passion for that. It is more likely some beastly wisdom that tells him that at last he has no hope of winning. That it is time to cut his losses, to slink off into high grass. Or is it some sober thought that pierces his wild brain, lacerating him in such a way that a hundred nightsticks could not? The thought of a woman who is waiting for him, perhaps? Or a child who, the next day and the week after that, will stare up at his terrible scars with a silent wonder that will shame him? For whatever reason, he is perfectly still.

It is four o'clock in the morning as I take the first stitch in his wound. At five-thirty, I snip each of the silks in his earlobes. He is released from his leg restrainers and pulled to a sitting position. The bandage on his head is a white turban. A single drop of blood in each earlobe, like a ruby. He is a maharajah.

The police return. All this time they have been drinking coffee with the nurses, the orderlies, other policemen, whomever. For over three hours the man and I have been alone in our devotion to the wound. "I have finished," I tell them. Roughly, they haul him from the stretcher and prod him toward the door. "Easy, easy," I call after them. And, to myself, if you hit him again ...

Even now, so many years later, this ancient rage of mine returns to peck among my dreams. I have only to close my eyes to see him again wielding his head and jaws, to hear once more those words at which the whole of his trussed body came hurtling toward me. How sorry I will always be. Not being able to make it up to him for that grin.

Laundry (*from* The Good Doctor)

Susan Onthank Mates

I was folding the baby's diapers—cloth, the kind they make now with a double thickness down the middle—and the phone rang. I was thinking and not thinking; just a second before, the baby had begun to scream that lightning-strike-of-hunger scream, so I was saying to him, wait just a minute let me smooth this crease, and he was shrieking a crescendo and the phone rang. While I was folding and talking to the baby underneath, I was thinking about whether, really, we could afford new bicycles for the girls, the used ones never seem to work quite right, surely it's not such an extravagance, new bikes, but if you've been to Toys 'R Us lately you realize this is a serious issue. On the other hand, I was the fourth child and never had anything new, so I understand that dream, that lust, for something smooth and shiny and unmarked and smelling like paint and not like old garage mildew. So I was thinking: maybe I should try to work another job, after all I am a doctor.

Hi, how are you, yes I'm Dr. Martin, pointing to the name tag that says Dr. Martin on the white coat that says doctor, doctor, doctor. So I hear you're having trouble breathing, pain in your side, a little nausea, the pills bothering you? So sorry to hear about your son, you must take care of yourself, no one can tell you for sure that you're going to die, it's a bad disease but there are always exceptions, god, hold my hand god, where in medical school did I miss that course on conviction THIS IS WHAT YOU SHOULD DO MR. DANTIO and me still folding diapers, patting them into squares warm and fresh from the dryer. I don't know Mr. Dantio, the cancer is all over your lungs those cells are eating you, collapsing you, deflating you, your X-ray looks like a drowned man, and each breath drives a spike of pain through your chest. Your wife sits in the corner and hates you and loves you and hates you. I see it in her eyes.

I don't know when can life end, myself I would rather die, but I'm a coward, always have been, I admire your ferocity—I can't help, I can't win this battle, slay the dragon, oh I want to be the hero now, I'll hold your hand Mr. Dantio. I'll watch when you scream and the water in your lungs bubbles up pink like cotton candy from your mouth and nostrils and I'll see the terror in your eyes as you try to pull a breath and your muscles contract and your ribs stand out like a skeleton and no air comes in and your children live three thousand miles away and hate you and love you and your wife is sobbing in the corner. I'm the doctor and I'm supposed to DO SOMETHING, the other doctors say why don't you scope him, biopsy him, give him a hit of chemo, cut him, needle him, anything but don't just let him die and Mr. Dantio I'm not just letting you die, it wasn't my decision, no one asked me should he live or die. But all I can do is watch, I will do that, I will watch even the very end when the air won't come and your fingers claw against the rails on the bed and you said no pain killers doctor, I want to see it coming and I said are you sure oh god.

Do you remember when we first met, and you complained that you itched, and it was flea bites and you had headaches, and it was because your wife yelled at you and you yelled at her, and you would call me in the middle of the night, and I would jump when the phone rang, my husband would groan and roll over in bed, one of the girls would start to cry, and the page operator said with a clothespin clipped on her nose Mr. Salvadore Dantio for you Dr. Martin and I would wake up and you would say, Doctor, that you doctor? Listen, I can't sleep for the itching. And there was nothing wrong with you and I hated you, but in the morning you would say, I'm sorry sorry, things get so bad in the middle of the night and what could I do but laugh, because it's true. The clinic didn't meet every day because I was supposed to do research and teach, I was the first woman doctor at the hospital, I was a role model, I was shiny and new and people whispered, so we met like lovers in the halls and in the lobbies really, you should try to come to your appointments, I said, Mr. Dantio I'll just squeeze you in today meet me on the second floor but next time KEEP YOUR APPOINTMENT and my friends said you'll never get ahead seeing patients in your research time like that, Mr. Dantio there was nothing wrong with you but your wife and your kids and your boss. You put your bony fingers over my hand and said how's a young girl like you a doctor? and I laughed, you drove me crazy. I'm forty Mr. Dantio forty and I don't know how to live and you finally did get something wrong with you Salvadore, you sure did.

The phone is ringing and the baby is crying and I just want to finish folding the diapers so I can balance them on top of the blue and yellow receiving blankets, which is why I didn't use bleach, which I should have because there is a large brown stain on one of the diapers. How did this happen to me? I swore never a housewife, never, never, I won't fall in that black hole, not me.

You grabbed my hand in that cold white room Mr. Dantio and you said I'm a fighter but only if there's a chance all these doctors want to cut me stick tubes in me I don't really understand I'm just a salesman now cake decorations, that's something I understand, you tell me what should I do. And I said I can't tell you that Mr. Dantio, Salvadore, I'm not you. And you said honey I need your help and you made your wife sobbing in the corner leave the room and you looked at me and I thought of you lying in the ICU with tubes in your mouth and arms and lungs and penis and nurses ripping the sheet off and turning your stiff blue body and brushing your hair and calling you sweetie while your blank brown eyes look up at the ceiling, you who never wanted a lady doctor who never wanted to be called sweetie, who always wanted to do the honey-sweetie calling and they're adjusting that tube in your penis and your hairless balls are flopping from side to side and no one even bothers to draw the curtain because your eyes are like mirrors: respirator, manometer, IV pump, electrocardiograph. Your heart keeps going on blip thump, blip thump and your lungs and your liver and your bone marrow filled with infection and your infection is so much like you that we are killing you both together and you asked me what should I do and I couldn't speak. I'm not god. You said well? And you looked out in the hall to make sure your wife wasn't coming in and we were running out of time and I stroked my nine months' pregnant belly and the baby kicked and I said studies show that sometimes if you have this biopsy and we treat you with antibiotics, antifungals, antivirals, you might live longer and you said don't tell me about studies tell me what you would do. And I said studies are important, this is the way doctors know what to do, it's scientific and more systematic than just one doctor's experience, I was good at that stuff even though women aren't supposed to be I knew studies and talked fast clear and incisive and honor society until then I was good at being a doctor. And you said please. I felt my breath clot up somewhere in my throat and I looked at your eyes your ferocious eyes and I said Mr. Dantio, Salvadore I would not do it, don't do it don't let them me do it to you no.

And I couldn't stop the tears, I kissed you and waddled out of the room and stood around the corner so your wife couldn't see me and I cried there right in the middle of the hall with my white coat split down the middle and my belly sticking out, the baby writhing like a snake making ripples in my navy-blue maternity dress with the little red bow on top. The surgeon came up to me, a young man, younger than me, so energetic and clean shaven and he said did you talk him into it? and he ignored the tears and the belly and the baby kicking so unprofessional and I said no.

No! he shouted at me and I said I know as a doctor I should have said do it but as a person I felt no no no and he looked at me and stared at me and finally said there is no difference between how I feel as a doctor and as a person and I saw him with his clean white coat buttoned down his flat front and his neat black hair actually he was a friend of mine I was looking up because he is taller and I said yes I can see that. I should have been angry or distant or something but I wasn't, it would be a lie to say I was—I was feeling no I'm no doctor, I never thickened and rooted and became "Doctor," something's wrong with me, I'm a lost pregnant woman with greasy hair and a discharge in my pants because the baby's coming and I don't know what to do because they never really helped me Plato Aristotle Kant Proust James all I know is this man Salvadore Dantio is dying and I can't do a thing.

I'm still folding the diapers, I have to do a load every day to keep up and the phone is ringing and all I could say Mr. Dantio was that I will be there when your pupils fix and dilate, when your jaw slackens and droops, I'll look though your teeth into the black cavern of your body, I'll smell the diarrhea as your bowels let loose with blood and shit, I'll stay Mr. Dantio, I won't look away. They lied to me about maternity leave and they said well we think you don't really want to be a doctor anyway, you must be conflicted to have a child, want to take two months off, no one sent me flowers they send flowers to all the wives of the doctors but no one sent me anything not even a card when I came back after three weeks still bleeding, I was the only woman doctor in the hospital anyway you never wanted a woman doctor Mr. Dantio, Salvadore, but in the end you looked straight into my eyes, Salvadore and I couldn't lie to you not to you.

I ran into your wife in the supermarket last week over the oranges and she saw me and began to cry and I put my arm around her and tried not to cry myself and she said to me you know when he died that Sunday I tried to call you but they jumped on him and pounded his chest and cut it open and squeezed his heart and he never wanted all of that and she cried and I wondered if she knew that they did it for me, the other doctors, because they knew I didn't want him to die so they couldn't watch him go so they cut him up for me they were embarrassed for me I cared so much I made a spectacle of myself standing in the hall crying. And when they took a piece of his lung, after he died, they found the infection, all I could think of was maybe I was wrong, maybe he could have lived longer if he'd had that biopsy, maybe I never learned this language right, medicine, I feel like I'm a visitor from some other world dressed up like a doctor but they can tell I'm not really one because in moments of great stress I revert to my native tongue. Mrs. Dantio wiped her eyes with the back of her hand and said is that the baby? And she looked at his smooth skin my little son and she smiled and touched the drool on his chin I laughed too.

He's still crying and I pick up the phone and someone says is this the lady of the house? and I don't know what to answer so I think but I still don't know so I hang up and reach for him, he's beginning to make those enunciated baby complaints. I pull up my shirt and my breasts hang out like a cow and just looking at him I feel that sweet pain contraction, the milk spurts and gets us wet. He makes snuffling noises he works his mouth searching for the nipple so I help him wham! he latch-es on and pulls and the milk is pouring out of both breasts now, I grab a diaper to hold over the other one but it's too late and we're drenched he and I a fecund shower. I know what this means: another load of laundry.

A Great Man

Frank O'Connor

Once when I was visiting a famous London hospital, I met the matron, Miss Fitzgerald, a small, good-looking woman of fifty. She was Irish, and we discussed acquaintances in common until I mentioned Dermot O'Malley, and then I realized that somehow or other I had said the wrong thing. The matron frowned and went away. A few minutes later she returned, smiling, and asked me to lunch in a way that, for some reason, reminded me of a girl asking a young fellow for the first time to her home. "You know, Dr. O'Malley was a great friend of my father," she said abruptly and then frowned again.

"Begor, I was," said O'Malley when I reported this to him later. "And I'll tell you a story about it, what's more." O'Malley is tall and gentle, and has a wife who is a pain in the neck, though he treats her with a consideration that I can only describe as angelic. "It was when I was a young doctor in Dublin, and my old professor, Dwyer, advised me to apply for a job in the hospital in Dooras. Now, you never heard of Dooras, but we all knew about it then, because that was in the days of Margaret's father, old Jim Fitzgerald, and he was known, all right.

"I met him a couple of nights later in a hotel in Kildare Street. He had come up to Dublin to attend a meeting of doctors. He was a man with piercing eyes and a long, hard face—more the face of a soldier than a doctor. The funny thing was his voice, which was rather high and piping and didn't seem to go at all with his manner.

" 'Dooras is no place for a young man who likes entertainment,' he said.

" 'Ah, I'm a country boy myself,' said I, 'so that wouldn't worry me. And of course, I know the hospital has a great reputation.'

" 'So I understand,' he said grimly. 'You see, O'Malley, I don't believe in all this centralization that's going on. I know it's all for the sake of equipment, and equipment is a good thing, too, but it's taking medicine away from where it belongs. One of these days, when their centralization breaks down, they'll find they haven't hospitals, doctors, or anything else.'

"By the time I'd left him, I'd as good as accepted the job, and it wasn't the job that interested me so much as the man. It could be that, my own father having been a bit of a waster, I'm attracted to men of strong character, and Fitzgerald was a fanatic. I liked that about him.

"Now, Dwyer had warned me that I'd find Dooras queer, and Dwyer knew the Dublin hospitals weren't up to much, but Dooras was dotty. It was an old hospital for infectious diseases that must have dated from about the time of the Famine, and Fitzgerald had got a small local committee to take it over. The first couple of days in it gave me the horrors, and it was weeks before I even began to see what Fitzgerald meant by it all. Then I did begin to see that in spite of all the drawbacks, it worked in a way bigger hospitals didn't work, and it was happy in a way that bigger hospitals are never happy. Everybody knew everybody else, and everybody was madly curious about everybody else, and if anybody ever gave a party, it wasn't something devised by the staff to entertain the patients; it was more likely to be the patients entertaining the staff.

"Partly this was because Margaret Fitzgerald, the woman you met in London, was the head nurse. I don't know what she's like now, and from all I can hear, she's a bit of a Tartar, but in those days she was a pretty little thing with an air of being more efficient than anybody ever was. Whenever you spoke to Margaret, she practically sprang to attention and clicked her heels, and if you were misguided enough to ask her for anything she hadn't handy, she gave you a demonstration of greyhound racing. And, of course, as you can see from the job she has now, she was a damn great nurse.

"But mainly the place worked because of Fitzgerald and his colleagues, the local doctors. Apart from him, none of them struck me as very brilliant, though he himself had a real respect for an old doctor called Pat Duane, a small, round, red-faced man with an old-fashioned choker collar and a wonderful soupy bedside manner. Pat looked as though some kind soul had let him to mature in a sherry cask till all the crude alcohol was drawn out of him. But they were all conscientious; they all listened to advice, even from me—and God knows I hadn't much to offer—and they all deferred in the most extraordinary way to Fitzgerald. Dwyer had described him to me as a remarkable man, and I was beginning to understand the full force of that, because I knew Irish small towns the way only a country boy knows them, and if those men weren't at one another's throats, fighting for every five-bob fee that could be picked up, it was due to his influence. I asked a doctor called MacCarthy about it one night and he invited me in for a drink. MacCarthy was a tall old poseur with a terrible passion for local history.

" 'Has it occurred to you that Fitzgerald may have given us back our self-respect, young man?' he asked in his pompous way.

" 'Our what?' I asked in genuine surprise. In those days it hadn't occurred to me that a man could at the same time be a show-box and be lacking in self-respect.

" 'Oh, come, O'Malley, come!' he said, sounding like the last Duke of Dooras. 'As a medical man you are more observant than you pretend. I presume you have met Dr. Duane?'

" 'I have. Yes,' said I.

" 'And it didn't occur to you that Dr. Duane was ever a victim of alcohol?' he went on portentously. 'You understand, of course, that I am not criticizing him. It isn't easy for the professional man in Ireland to maintain his standards of behavior. Fitzgerald has a considerable respect for Dr. Duane's judgment—quite justified, I may add, quite justified. But at any rate, in a very short time Pat eased off on the drink, and even began to read the medical journals again. Now Fitzgerald has him in the hollow of his hand. We all like to feel we are of some use to humanity— even the poor general practitioner.... But you saw it all for yourself, of course. You are merely trying to pump a poor country doctor.'

"Fitzgerald was not pretentious. He liked me to drop in on him when I had an hour to spare, and I went to his house every week for dinner. He lived in an old, uncomfortable family house a couple of miles out on the bay. Normally, he was cold, concentrated, and irritable, but when he had a few drinks in he got melancholy, and this for some reason caused him to be indiscreet and say dirty things about his committee and even about the other doctors. 'The most interesting thing about MacCarthy,' he said to me once, 'is that he's the seventh son of a seventh son, and so he can diagnose a case without seeing the patient at all. It leaves him a lot of spare time for local history.' I suspected he made the same sort of dirty remarks about me, and that secretly the man had no faith in anyone but himself. I told him so, and I think he enjoyed it. Like all shy men he liked to be insulted in a broad masculine way, and one night when I called him a flaming egotist, he grunted like an old dog when you tickle him and said, 'Drink makes you very offensive, O'Malley. Have some more!'

"It wasn't so much that he was an egotist (though he was) as that he had a pernickety sense of responsibility, and whenever he hadn't a case to worry over, he could always find some equivalent of a fatal disease in the hospital—a porter who was too cheeky or a nurse who made too free with the men patients—and he took it all personally and on a very high level of suffering. He would sulk and snap at Margaret for days over some trifle that didn't matter to anyone, and finally reduce her to tears. At the same time, I suppose it was part of the atmosphere of seriousness he had created about the makeshift hospital, and it kept us all on our toes. Medicine was his life, and his gossip was shop. Duane or MacCarthy or some other local doctor would drop in of an evening to discuss a case—which by some process I never was able to fathom had become Fitzgerald's case—and over the drinks he would grow gloomier and gloomier about our ignorance till at last, without a word to any of us, he got up and telephoned some Dublin specialist he knew. It was part of the man's shyness that he only did it when he was partly drunk and could pretend that instead of asking a favor he was conferring one. Several times I watched that scene with amusement. It was all carefully calculated, because if he hadn't had enough to drink he lacked the brass and became apologetic, whereas if he had had one drink too much he could not describe what it was about the case that really worried him. Not that he rated a specialist's knowledge any higher than ours, but it seemed the best he could do, and if that didn't satisfy him, he ordered the specialist down, even when it meant footing the bill himself. It was only then I began to realize the respect that Dublin specialists had for him, because Dwyer, who was a terrified little man and hated to leave home for fear of what might happen him in out-of-the-way places like Cork and Belfast, would only give out a gentle moan about coming to Dooras. No wonder Duane and MacCarthy swore by him, even if for so much of the time they, like myself, thought him a nuisance.

"Margaret was a second edition of himself, though in her the sense of responsibility conflicted with everything feminine in her till it became a joke. She was small. She was pretty, with one of those miniature faces that seem to have been reduced until every coarse line has been refined in them. She moved at twice the normal speed and was forever fussing and bossing and wheedling, till one of the nurses would lose her temper and say, 'Ah, Margaret, will you for God's sake give us time to breathe!' That sort of impertinence would make Margaret scowl, shrug, and go off somewhere else, but her sulks never lasted, as her father's did. The feminine side of her wouldn't sustain them.

"I remember one night when all hell broke loose in the wards, as it usually does in any hospital once a month. Half a dozen patients decided to die all together, and I was called out of bed. Margaret and the other nurse on night duty, Joan Henderson, had brewed themselves a pot of tea in the kitchen, and they were scurrying round with a mug or a bit of seedcake in their hands. I was giving an injection to one of my patients, who should have been ready for discharge. In the next bed was a dying old mountainy man who had nothing in particular wrong with him except old age and a broken heart. I suddenly looked up from what I was doing and saw he had come out of coma and was staring at Margaret, who was standing at the other side of the bed from me, 'nibbling the bit of cake over which she had been interrupted. She started when she saw him staring at the cake, because she knew what her father would say if ever he heard that she was eating in the wards. Then she gave a broad grin and said in a country accent, 'Johnny, would 'oo like a bit of seedcake?' and held it to his lips. He hesitated and then began to nibble, too, and then his tongue came out and licked round his mouth, and somehow I knew he was saved. 'Tay, Johnny,' she said mockingly. 'Thot's what 'oo wants now, isn't it?' And that morning as I went through the wards, my own patient was dead but old Johnny was sitting up, ready for another ten years of the world's hardship. That's nursing.

"Margaret lived in such a pitch of nervous energy that every few weeks she fell ill. 'I keep telling that damn girl to take it easy,' her father would say with a scowl at me, but any time there was the least indication that Margaret was taking it easy, he started to air his sufferings with the anguish of an elephant. She was a girl with a real sense of service, and at one time had tried to join a nursing order in Africa, but dropped it because of his hatred for all nursing orders. In itself this was funny, because Margaret was a liberal Catholic who, like St. Teresa, was 'for the Moors, and martyrdom' but never worried her head about human weaknesses and made no more of an illegitimate baby than if she had them herself every Wednesday, while he was an old-fashioned Catholic and full of obscure prejudices. At the same time, he felt that the religious orders were leaving Ireland without nurses—not that he thought so much of nurses!

" 'And I suppose nuns can't be nurses?' Margaret would ask with a contemptuous shrug.

" 'How can they?' he would say, in his shrillest voice. The business of religion is with the soul, not the body. My business is with the body. When I'm done with it, the nuns can have it—Or anyone else, for that matter.'

"'And why not the soul and the body?' Margaret would ask in her pertest tone.

" 'Because you can't serve two masters, girl.'

"'Pooh!' Margaret would say with another shrug. 'You can't serve one Siamese twin, either.'

"As often as I went to dinner in that house, there was hardly a meal without an argument. Sometimes it was about no more than the amount of whiskey he drank. Margaret hated drink, and watched every drop he poured in his glass, so that often, just to spite her, he went on to knock himself out. I used to think that she might have known her father was a man who couldn't resist a challenge. She was as censorious as he was, but she had a pertness and awkwardness that a man rarely has, and suddenly, out of the blue, would come some piece of impertinence that plunged him into gloom and made her cringe away to her bedroom, ready for tears. He and I would go into the big front room, overlooking Dooras Bay, and without a glance at the view he would splash enormous tasheens of whiskey into our glasses, just to indicate how little he cared for her, and say in a shrill, complaining voice, 'I ruined that girl, O'Malley. I know I did. If her mother was alive, she wouldn't talk to me that way.'

"Generally, they gave the impression of two people who hated one another with a passionate intensity, but I knew well that he was crazy about her. He always brought her back something from his trips to Dublin or Cork and once when I was with him, he casually wasted my whole afternoon looking for something nice for her. It never occurred to him that I might have anything else to do. But he could also be thoughtful; for once when for a full week he had been so intolerable that I could scarcely bring myself to answer him he grinned and said, 'I know exactly what you think of me, O'Malley. You think I'm an old slave driver.'

" 'Not exactly,' I said, giving him tit for tat. 'Just an old whoor!'

"At this, he gave a great gaffaw and handed me a silver cigarette case, which I knew he must have bought for me in town the previous day, and added sneeringly, 'Now, don't you be going round saying your work is quite unappreciated.'

"'Did I really say that?' I asked, still keeping my end up, even though there was something familiar about the sentiment.

" 'Or if you do, say it over the loudspeaker. Remember, O'Malley, I hear everything. ' And the worst of it was, he did!

"Then, one night, when my year's engagement was nearly ended, I went to his house for dinner. That night there was no quarrelling, and he and I sat on in the front room, drinking and admiring the view. I should have known there was something wrong, because for once he didn't talk shop. He talked about almost everything else, and all the time he was knocking back whiskey in a way I knew I could never keep pace with. When it grew dark, he said with an air of surprise, 'O'Malley, I'm a bit tight. I think we'd better go for a stroll and clear our heads.'

"We strolled up the avenue of rhododendrons to the gate and turned left up the hill. It was a wild, rocky bit of country, stopped dead by the roadway and then cascading merrily down the little fields to the bay. There was still a coppery light in the sky, and the reflection of a bon-fire on one of the islands, like a pendulum, in the water. The road fell again, between demesne walls and ruined gateways where the last of the old gentry lived, and I was touched—partly, I suppose, by all the whiskey, but partly by the place itself.

" 'I'll regret this place when I leave it,' I said.

"'Oh, no, you won't,' he snapped back at me. 'This is no place for young people.'

" 'I fancy it might be a very pleasant memory if you were in the East End of London,' said I.

" 'It might,' said Fitzgerald, 'if you were quite sure you wouldn't have to go back to it. That's what worries me about Margaret.'

"I had never noticed him worrying very much about Margaret—or anyone else, for that matter—so I took it as merely a matter of form.

" 'Margaret seems to do very well in it,' I said.

" 'It's no place for Margaret,' he said sharply. 'People need friends of their own age and ideas old men like myself can't supply. It's largely my fault for letting her come back here at all. I made this place too much of my life, and that's all right for a man, but it's not good enough for a high-spirited girl like that.'

" 'But doesn't Margaret have friends here?' I asked, trying to comfort him.

" 'She has friends enough, but not of her own age,' he said. 'She's too mature for the girls here that are her own age. Not that I ever cared much for her friends from Dublin,' he added shortly. 'They struck me as a lot of show-boxes. I don't like those intellectual Catholics, talking to me about St. Thomas Aquinas. I never read St. Thomas Aquinas, and from all I can hear I haven't missed much. But young people have to make their own mistakes. All the men around here seem to want is some good-natured cow who'll agree to everything they say, and because she argues with them they think she's pert and knowing. Well, she is pert, and she is knowing—I realize that as well as anybody. But there's more than that to her. They'd have said the same about me, only I proved to them that I knew what I was doing.'

"Suddenly I began to realize what he was saying, and I was frightened out of my wits. I said to myself that it was impossible, that a man like Fitzgerald could never mean a thing like that, but at the same time I felt that he did mean it, and that it had been in his mind from the first night he met me. I muttered something about her having more chances in Dublin.

" 'That's the trouble,' he said. 'She didn't know what she was letting herself in for when she came back here, and no more did I. Now she won't leave, because I'd be here on my own, and I know I wouldn't like it, but still I have my work to do, and for a man that's enough. I like pitting my wits against parish priests and county councillors and nuns. Besides, when you reach my age you realize that you could have worse, and they'll let me have my own way for the time I have left me. But I haven't so long to live, and when I die, they'll have some champion footballer running the place, and Margaret will be taking orders from the nuns. She thinks now that she won't mind, but she won't do it for long. I know the girl. She ought to marry, and then she'd have to go wherever her husband took her.'

" 'But you don't really think the hospital will go to pieces like that?' I asked, pretending to be deeply concerned but really only trying to head Fitzgerald off the subject he seemed to have on his mind. 'I mean, don't you think Duane and MacCarthy will hold it together?'

" 'How can they?' he asked querulously. 'It's not their life, the way it's been mine. I don't mean they won't do their best, but the place will go to pieces just the same. It's a queer feeling, Dermot, when you come to the end of your time and realize that nothing in the world outlasts the man that made it.'

"That sentence was almost snapped at me, out of the side of his mouth; and yet it sounded like a cry of pain—maybe because he'd used my Christian name for the first time. He was not a man to use Christian names. I didn't know what to say.

" 'Of course, I should have had a son to pass on my responsibilities to,' he added wonderingly. 'I'm not any good with girls. I dare say that was why I liked you, the first time we met—because I might have had a son like you.'

"Then I couldn't bear it any longer, and it broke from me. 'And it wasn't all on one side!'

" 'I guessed that. In certain ways we're not so unlike. And that's what I really wanted to say to you before you go. If ever you and Margaret got to care for one another, it would mean a lot to me. She won't have much, but she'll never be a burden on anybody, and if ever she marries, she'll make a good wife.'

"It was the most embarrassing moment of my life—and mind, it wasn't embarrassing just because I was being asked to marry a nice girl I'd never given a thought to. I'm a country boy, and I knew all about 'made' matches by the time I was seventeen, and I never had anything but contempt for the snobs that pretend to despise them. Damn good matches the most of them are, and a thousand times better than the sort you see nowadays that seem to be made up out of novelettes or moving pictures! Still and all, it's different when it comes to your own turn. I suppose it's only at a moment like that you realize you're just as silly as any little servant girl. But it wasn't only that. It was because I was being proposed to by a great man, a fellow I'd looked up to in a way I never looked up to my own father, and I couldn't do the little thing he wanted me to do. I muttered some nonsense about never having been able to think about marriage—as if there ever was a young fellow that hadn't thought about it every night in his life!—and he saw how upset I was and squeezed my arm.

" 'What did I tell you?' he said. 'I knew I was drunk, and if she ever gets to hear what I said to you, she'll cut me in little bits.'

"And that tone of his broke my heart. I don't even know if you'll understand what I mean, but all I felt was grief to think a great man who'd brought life to a place where life never was before would have to ask a favor of me, and me not to be able to grant it. Because all the time I wanted to be cool and suave and say of course I'd marry his daughter, just to show the way I felt about himself, and I was too much of a coward to do it. In one way, it seemed so impossible, and in another it seemed such a small thing.

"Of course, we never resumed the conversation, but that didn't make it any easier, because it wasn't only between myself and him; it was between me and Margaret. The moment I had time to think of it, I knew Fitzgerald was too much a gentleman to have said anything to me without first making sure that she'd have me.

"Well, you know the rest yourself. When he died, things happened exactly the way he'd prophesied; a local footballer got his job, and the nuns took over the nursing, and there isn't a Dublin doctor under fifty that could even tell you where Dooras is. Fitzgerald was right. Nothing in the world outlasts a man. Margaret, of course, has a great reputation, and I'm told on the best authority that there isn't a doctor in St. Dorothy's she hasn't put the fear of God into so I suppose it's just as well that she never got the opportunity to put it into me. Or don't you agree?"

I didn't, of course, as O'Malley well knew. Anyway, he could hardly have done much worse for himself. And I had met Margaret, and I had seen her autocratic airs, but they hadn't disturbed me much. She was just doing it on temperament, rather than technique—a very Irish way, and probably not so unlike her father's. I knew I didn't have to tell O'Malley that. He was a gentleman himself, and his only reason for telling me the story was that already, with the wisdom that comes of age, he had begun to wonder whether he had not missed something in missing Margaret Fitzgerald. I knew that he had.

from Life On The Mississippi

Mark Twain

Now when I had mastered the language of this water and had come to know every trifling feature that bordered the great river as familiarly as I knew the letters of the alphabet, I had made a valuable acquisition. But I had lost something, too. I had lost something which could never be restored to me while I lived. All the grace, the beauty, the poetry had gone out of the majestic river! I still keep in mind a certain wonderful sunset which I witnessed when steamboating was new to me. A broad expanse of the river was turned to blood; in the middle distance the red hue brightened into gold, through which a solitary log came floating, black and conspicuous; in one place a long, slanting mark lay sparkling upon the water; in another the surface was broken by boiling, tumbling rings, that were as many-tinted as an opal; where the ruddy flush was faintest, was a smooth spot that was covered with graceful circles and radiating lines, ever so delicately traced; the shore on our left was densely wooded, and the somber shadow that fell from this forest was broken in one place by a long, ruffled trail that shone like silver; and high above the forest wall a clean-stemmed dead tree waved a single leafy bough that glowed like a flame in the unobstructed splendor that was flowing from the sun. There were graceful curves, reflected images, woody heights, soft distances; and over the whole scene, far and near, the dissolving lights drifted steadily, enriching it, every passing moment, with new marvels of coloring.

I stood like one bewitched. I drank it in, in a speechless rapture. The world was new to me, and I had never seen anything like this at home. But as I have said, a day came when I began to cease from noting the glories and the charms which the moon and the sun and the twilight wrought upon the river's face; another day came when I ceased altogether to note them. Then, if that sunset scene had been repeated, I should have looked upon it without rapture, and should have commented upon it, inwardly, after this fashion: This sun means that we are going to have wind to-morrow; that floating log means that the river is rising, small thanks to it; that slanting mark on the water refers to a bluff reef which is going to kill somebody's steamboat one of these nights, if it keeps on stretching out like that; those tumbling 'boils' show a dissolving bar and a changing channel there; the lines and circles in the slick water over yonder are a warning that that troublesome place is shoaling up dangerously; that silver streak in the shadow of the forest is the 'break' from a new snag, and he has located himself in the very best place he could have found to fish for steamboats; that tall dead tree, with a single living branch, is not going to last long, and then how is a body ever going to get through this blind place at night without the friendly old landmark.

No, the romance and the beauty were all gone from the river. All the value any feature of it had for me now was the amount of usefulness it could furnish toward compassing the safe piloting of a steamboat. Since those days, I have pitied doctors from my heart. What does the lovely flush in a beauty's cheek mean to a doctor but a 'break' that ripples above some deadly disease. Are not all her visible charms sown thick with what are to him the signs and symbols of hidden decay? Does he ever see her beauty at all, or doesn't he simply view her professionally, and comment upon her unwholesome condition all to himself? And doesn't he sometimes wonder whether he has gained most or lost most by learning his trade?

Death in the Open

Lewis Thomas

Most of the dead animals you see on highways near the cities are dogs, a few cats. Out in the country-side, the forms and coloring of the dead are strange; these are the wild creatures. Seen from a car window they appear as fragments, evoking memories of wood-chucks, badgers, skunks, voles, snakes, sometimes the mysterious wreckage of a deer.

It is always a queer shock, part a sudden upwelling of grief, part unaccountable amazement. It is simply astounding to see an animal dead on a highway. The outrage is more than just the location; it is the impropriety of such visible death, anywhere. You do not expect to see dead animals in the open. It is the nature of animals to die alone, off somewhere, hidden. It is wrong to see them lying out on the highway; it is wrong to see them anywhere.

Everything in the world dies, but we only know about it as a kind of abstraction. If you stand in a meadow, at the edge of a hillside, and look around carefully, almost everything you can catch sight of is in the process of dying, and most things will be dead long before you are. If it were not for the constant renewal and replacement going on before your eyes, the whole place would turn to stone and sand under your feet.

There are some creatures that do not seem to die at all; they simply vanish totally into their own progeny. Single cells do this. The cell becomes two, then four, and so on, and after a while the last trace is gone. It cannot be seen as death; barring mutation, the descendants are simply the first cell, living all over again. The cycles of the slime mold have episodes that seem as conclusive as death, but the withered slug, with its stalk and fruiting body, is plainly the transient tissue of a developing animal; the free-swimming amebocytes use this organ collectively in order to produce more of themselves.

There are said to be a billion billion insects on the earth at any moment, most of them with very short life expectancies by our standards. Someone has estimated that there are 25 million assorted insects hanging in the air over every temperate square mile, in a column extending upward for thousands of feet, drifting through the layers of the atmosphere like plankton. They are dying steadily, some by being eaten, some just dropping in their tracks, tons of them around the earth, disintegrating as they die, invisibly.

Who ever sees dead birds, in anything like the huge numbers stipulated by the certainty of the death of all birds? A dead bird is an incongruity, more startling than an unexpected live bird, sure evidence to the human mind that something has gone wrong. Birds do their dying off somewhere, behind things, under things, never on the wing.

Animals seem to have an instinct for performing death alone, hidden. Even the largest most conspicuous ones find ways to conceal themselves in time. If an elephant missteps and dies in an open place, the herd will not leave him there; the others will pick him up and carry the body from place to place, finally putting it down in some inexplicably suitable location. When elephants encounter the skeleton of an elephant out in the open, they methodically take up each of the bones and distribute them, in a ponderous ceremony, over neighboring acres.

It is a natural marvel. All of the life on the earth dies, all of the time, in the same volume as the new life that dazzles us each morning, each spring. All we see of this is the odd stump, the fly struggling on the porch floor of the summer house in October, the fragment on the highway. I have lived all my life with an embarrassment of squirrels in my backyard, they are all over the place, all year long, and I have never seen, anywhere, a dead squirrel.

I suppose it is just as well. If the earth were otherwise, and all the dying were done in the open, with the dead there to be looked at, we would never have it out of our minds. We can forget about it much of the time, or think of it as an accident to be avoided, somehow. But it does make the process of dying seem more exceptional than it really is, and harder to engage in at the times when we must ourselves engage.

In our way, we conform as best we can to the rest of nature. The obituary pages tell us of the news that we are dying away, while the birth announcements in finer print, off at the side of the page, inform us of our replacements, but we get no grasp from this of the enormity of scale. There are 3 billion of us on the earth, and all 3 billion must be dead, on a schedule, within this lifetime. The vast mortality, involving something over 50 million of us each year, takes place in relative secrecy. WE can only really know of the deaths in our households, or among our friends. These, detached in our minds from all the rest, we take to be unnatural events, anomalies, outrages. We speak of our own dead in low voices; struck down, we say, as though visible death can only occur for cause, by disease or violence, avoidably. We send off for flowers, grieve, make ceremonies, scatter bones, unaware of the rest of the 3 billion on the same schedule. All of that immense mass of flesh and bone and consciousness will disappear by absorption into the earth, without recognition by the transient survivors.

Less than a half a century form now, our replacements will have more than doubled the numbers. It is hard to see how we can continue to keep the secret, with such multitudes doing the dying. We will have to give up on the notion that death is catastrophe, or detestable, or avoidable, or even strange. We will need to learn more about the cycling of life in the rest of the system, and about our connection to the process. Everything that comes alive seems to be in trade for something that dies, cell for cell. There might be some comfort in the recognition of synchrony, in the information that we all go down together, in the best of company.

A Favorite Charity That Won't Accept Donations

Abigail Zuger

Every day, as usual in this season of charity, pleas for money arrive in the mail. Thumbing through them, I realize all over again that there is only one good cause I have any real enthusiasm for, and she is not accepting donations.

She came in to see me last month, after a long hiatus. Frankly, I thought she was dead. But no, she had simply fallen through the cracks, as we like to term all the various ways people can get lost in our so-called system.

With an income right at the Medicaid cutoff, so that some months they have health insurance and some months they don't, they teeter at the edge of one crack. With a half-dozen chronic medical problems that are too stable for the hospital, but too misery-making to leave them much enthusiasm for getting out of bed, they straddle another. With a telephone that keeps getting cut off for lack of payment they wander along a third.

And with a steely determination to take nothing from anyone you risk toppling into the most dangerous one of all, the crack that will swallow them up and never let them go.

Pretty and petite on the outside, this woman has the granite soul of a pioneer or a patriarch. All she wants is to go it on her own.

All I want is to write her a check.

She is every good cause built into one. Once a perfectly ordinary working citizen, she has had a run of the worst luck imaginable. Her husband is dead, and her career is a vague memory from the 1990s, as is the last day she felt really well. At times there is no food in the house. Her pain is better some days than others but never goes away. Her bathroom ceiling is falling in.

With all this, she is dignified, well groomed, cheerful and polite. So are her children, both heading for college on some unclear combination of grit and magic. Others in her position demand the moon. She tells us she just needs a few weeks to get herself together and she'll start looking for work, so thanks so much, but the usual resources we muster in cases like hers, from disability payments to home-delivered meals, won't be necessary.

Occasionally, health and money have little to do with each other. In her case, the relation could not be clearer. If she keeps on her present trajectory, she'll be lucky to live another year. Were I to concentrate all my charitable giving on her for a while, I bet I could buy her decades.

The idea is preposterous. Even if she would take money, doctors simply do not give it. We give our time and skills; we give out tests, advice and little pieces of paper written in Latin. The various ethical codes that guide our behavior go into some detail about when and from whom we should not accept money. They never bother to discuss when we should not give it out, because, in theory, we never do.

The theory is reasonable: the relationship with patients is complex enough without adding yet another layer of guilt, obligation and responsibility.

But the practice is something else again. Some situations simply leave no alternative but to give. A few years ago, the head of a kidney transplant program in Illinois found herself in such a situation; she wound up giving a patient one of her kidneys. Similarly, if less heroically, it is not possible to work among the destitute without scrounging around in your pocket from time to time.

A few dollars for lunch, a twenty to last the weekend: usually all is repaid promptly, with thanks. Once a patient vanished with the loan, missing appointments for almost a year. When she finally showed up again, the first thing she did was press $20 into my hand. "Couldn't come back without it," she said.

I felt like a fool, having managed to completely undermine her medical care with my charity.

But despite this instructive lesson, I still indulge in fantasies of saving my needy patient with a solid hunk of cash, an anonymous check — enough to buy her food and transportation; expert, consistent medical care; a few treats; and a little something in the bank.

It is an idiotic fantasy. But perhaps no more idiotic than for me to write out checks this month that will cover an infinitesimal fraction of some giant charity's overhead. No more idiotic than for me to labor over Latin incantations on little scraps of paper in the illusion that they alone will make a difference in my patient's health and life.

from Pierre Curie

Marie Curie

A nd now, let us glance at this narrative as a whole, in which I have attempted to evoke the image of a man who, inflexibly devoted to the service of his ideal, honored humanity by an existence lived in silence, in the simple grandeur of his genius and his character. He had the faith of those who open new ways. He knew that he had a high mission to fulfil and the mystic dream of his youth pushed him invincibly beyond the usual path of life into a way which he called anti-natural because it signified the renunciation of the pleasures of life. Nevertheless, he resolutely subordinated his thoughts and desires to this dream, adapting himself to it and identifying himself with it more and more completely. Believing only in the pacific might of science and of reason, he lived for the search of truth. Without prejudice or parti pris, he carried the same loyalty into his study of things that he used in his understanding of other men and of himself. Detached from every common passion, seeking neither supremacy nor honors, he had no enemies, even though the effort he had achieved in the control of himself had made of him one of those elect whom we find in advance of their time in all the epochs of civilization. Like them he was able to exercise a profound influence merely by the radiation of his inner strength.

It is useful to learn how much sacrifice such a life represents. The life of a great scientist in his laboratory is not, as many may think, a peaceful idyll. More often it is a bitter battle with things, with one's surroundings, and above all with oneself. A great discovery does not leap completely achieved from the brain of the scientist, as Minerva sprang, all panoplied, from the head of Jupiter; it is the fruit of accumulated preliminary work. Between the days of fecund productivity are inserted days of uncertainty when nothing seems to succeed, and when even matter itself seems hostile; and it is then that one must hold out against discouragement. Thus without ever forsaking his inexhaustible patience, Pierre Curie used sometimes to say to me: "It is nevertheless hard, this life that we have chosen."

For the admirable gift of himself, and for the magnificent service he renders humanity, what reward does our society offer the scientist? Have these servants of an idea the necessary means of work? Have they an assured existence, sheltered from care? The example of Pierre Curie, and of others, shows that they have none of these things; and that more often, before they can secure possible working conditions, they have to exhaust their youth and their powers in daily anxieties. Our society, in which reigns an eager desire for riches and luxury, does not understand the value of science. It does not realize that science is a most precious part of its moral patrimony. Nor does it take sufficient cognizance of the fact that science is at the base of all the progress that lightens the burden of life and lessens its suffering. Neither public powers nor private generosity actually accord to science and to scientists the support and the subsidies indispensable to fully effective work.

I invoke, in closing, the admirable pleading of Pasteur:

"If the conquests useful for humanity touch your heart, if you are overwhelmed before the astonishing results of electric telegraphy, of the daguerrotype, of anesthesia, and of other wonderful discoveries, if you are jealous of the part your country may claim in the spreading of these marvelous things, take an interest, I beg of you, in those sacred places to which we give the expressive name of laboratories.Demand that they be multiplied and ornamented, for these are the temples of the future, of wealth, and of well-being. It is in them that humanity grows, fortifies itself, and becomes better. There it may learn to read in the works of nature the story of progress and of universal harmony, even while its own creations are too often those of barbarism, fanaticism, and destruction."

May this truth be widely spread, and deeply penetrate public opinion, that the future may be less hard for the pioneers who must open up new domains for the general good of humanity.

A Doctor's Visit

Anton Chekhov

The Professor received a telegram from the Lyalikovs' factory; he was asked to come as quickly as possible. The daughter of some Madame Lyalikov, apparently the owner of the factory, was ill, and that was all that one could make out of the long, incoherent telegram. And the Professor did not go himself, but sent instead his assistant, Korolyov.

It was two stations from Moscow, and there was a drive of three miles from the station. A carriage with three horses had been sent to the station to meet Korolyov; the coachman wore a hat with a peacock's feather on it, and answered every question in a loud voice like a soldier: "No, sir!" "Certainly, sir!"

It was Saturday evening; the sun was setting, the workpeople were coming in crowds from the factory to the station, and they bowed to the carriage in which Korolyov was driving. And he was charmed with the evening, the farmhouses and villas on the road, and the birch-trees, and the quiet atmosphere all around, when the fields and woods and the sun seemed preparing, like the workpeople now on the eve of the holiday, to rest, and perhaps to pray. . . .

He was born and had grown up in Moscow; he did not know the country, and he had never taken any interest in factories, or been inside one, but he had happened to read about factories, and had been in the houses of manufacturers and had talked to them; and whenever he saw a factory far or near, he always thought how quiet and peaceable it was outside, but within there was always sure to be impenetrable ignorance and dull egoism on the side of the owners, wearisome, unhealthy toil on the side of the workpeople, squabbling, vermin, vodka. And now when the workpeople timidly and respectfully made way for the carriage, in their faces, their caps, their walk, he read physical impurity, drunkenness, nervous exhaustion, bewilderment.

They drove in at the factory gates. On each side he caught glimpses of the little houses of workpeople, of the faces of women, of quilts and linen on the railings. "Look out!" shouted the coachman, not pulling up the horses. It was a wide courtyard without grass, with five immense blocks of buildings with tall chimneys a little distance one from another, warehouses and barracks, and over everything a sort of grey powder as though from dust. Here and there, like oases in the desert, there were pitiful gardens, and the green and red roofs of the houses in which the managers and clerks lived. The coachman suddenly pulled up the horses, and the carriage stopped at the house, which had been newly painted grey; here was a flower garden, with a lilac bush covered with dust, and on the yellow steps at the front door there was a strong smell of paint.

"Please come in, doctor," said women's voices in the passage and the entry, and at the same time he heard sighs and whisperings. "Pray walk in. . . . We've been expecting you so long. . . we're in real trouble. Here, this way."

Madame Lyalikov—a stout elderly lady wearing a black silk dress with fashionable sleeves, but, judging from her face, a simple uneducated woman—looked at the doctor in a flutter, and could not bring herself to hold out her hand to him; she did not dare. Beside her stood a personage with short hair and a pince-nez; she was wearing a blouse of many colours, and was very thin and no longer young. The servants called her Christina Dmitryevna, and Korolyov guessed that this was the governess. Probably, as the person of most education in the house, she had been charged to meet and receive the doctor, for she began immediately, in great haste, stating the causes of the illness, giving trivial and tiresome details, but without saying who was ill or what was the matter.

The doctor and the governess were sitting talking while the lady of the house stood motionless at the door, waiting. From the conversation Korolyov learned that the patient was Madame Lyalikov's only daughter and heiress, a girl of twenty, called Liza; she had been ill for a long time, and had consulted various doctors, and the previous night she had suffered till morning from such violent palpitations of the heart, that no one in the house had slept, and they had been afraid she might die.

"She has been, one may say, ailing from a child," said Christina Dmitryevna in a sing-song voice, continually wiping her lips with her hand. "The doctors say it is nerves; when she was a little girl she was scrofulous, and the doctors drove it inwards, so I think it may be due to that."

They went to see the invalid. Fully grown up, big and tall, but ugly like her mother, with the same little eyes and disproportionate breadth of the lower part of the face, lying with her hair in disorder, muffled up to the chin, she made upon Korolyov at the first minute the impression of a poor, destitute creature, sheltered and cared for here out of charity, and he could hardly believe that this was the heiress of the five huge buildings.

"I am the doctor come to see you," said Korolyov. "Good evening."

He mentioned his name and pressed her hand, a large, cold, ugly hand; she sat up, and, evidently accustomed to doctors, let herself be sounded, without showing the least concern that her shoulders and chest were uncovered.

"I have palpitations of the heart," she said, "It was so awful all night. . . . I almost died of fright! Do give me something."

"I will, I will; don't worry yourself."

Korolyov examined her and shrugged his shoulders.

"The heart is all right," he said; "it's all going on satisfactorily; everything is in good order. Your nerves must have been playing pranks a little, but that's so common. The attack is over by now, one must suppose; lie down and go to sleep."

At that moment a lamp was brought into the bed-room. The patient screwed up her eyes at the light, then suddenly put her hands to her head and broke into sobs. And the impression of a destitute, ugly creature vanished, and Korolyov no longer noticed the little eyes or the heavy development of the lower part of the face. He saw a soft, suffering expression which was intelligent and touching: she seemed to him altogether graceful, feminine, and simple; and he longed to soothe her, not with drugs, not with advice, but with simple, kindly words. Her mother put her arms round her head and hugged her. What despair, what grief was in the old woman's face! She, her mother, had reared her and brought her up, spared nothing, and devoted her whole life to having her daughter taught French, dancing, music: had engaged a dozen teachers for her; had consulted the best doctors, kept a governess. And now she could not make out the reason of these tears, why there was all this misery, she could not understand, and was bewildered; and she had a guilty, agitated, despairing expression, as though she had omitted something very important, had left something undone, had neglected to call in somebody—and whom, she did not know.

"Lizanka, you are crying again . . . again," she said, hugging her daughter to her. "My own, my darling, my child, tell me what it is! Have pity on me! Tell me."

Both wept bitterly. Korolyov sat down on the side of the bed and took Liza's hand.

"Come, give over; it's no use crying," he said kindly. "Why, there is nothing in the world that is worth those tears. Come, we won't cry; that's no good. . . ."

And inwardly he thought:

"It's high time she was married. . . ."

"Our doctor at the factory gave her kalibromati," said the governess, "but I notice it only makes her worse. I should have thought that if she is given anything for the heart it ought to be drops. . . . I forget the name. . . . Convallaria, isn't it?"

And there followed all sorts of details. She interrupted the doctor, preventing his speaking, and there was a look of effort on her face, as though she supposed that, as the woman of most education in the house, she was duty bound to keep up a conversation with the doctor, and on no other subject but medicine.

Korolyov felt bored.

"I find nothing special the matter," he said, addressing the mother as he went out of the bedroom. "If your daughter is being attended by the factory doctor, let him go on attending her. The treatment so far has been perfectly correct, and I see no reason for changing your doctor. Why change? It's such an ordinary trouble; there's nothing seriously wrong."

He spoke deliberately as he put on his gloves, while Madame Lyalikov stood without moving, and looked at him with her tearful eyes.

"I have half an hour to catch the ten o'clock train," he said. "I hope I am not too late."

"And can't you stay?" she asked, and tears trickled down her cheeks again. "I am ashamed to trouble you, but if you would be so good. . . . For God's sake," she went on in an undertone, glancing towards the door, "do stay to-night with us! She is all I have . . . my only daughter. . . . She frightened me last night; I can't get over it. . . . Don't go away, for goodness' sake! . . ."

He wanted to tell her that he had a great deal of work in Moscow, that his family were expecting him home; it was disagreeable to him to spend the evening and the whole night in a strange house quite needlessly; but he looked at her face, heaved a sigh, and began taking off his gloves without a word.

All the lamps and candles were lighted in his honour in the drawing-room and the dining-room. He sat down at the piano and began turning over the music. Then he looked at the pictures on the walls, at the portraits. The pictures, oil-paintings in gold frames, were views of the Crimea—a stormy sea with a ship, a Catholic monk with a wineglass; they were all dull, smooth daubs, with no trace of talent in them. There was not a single good-looking face among the portraits, nothing but broad cheekbones and astonished-looking eyes. Lyalikov, Liza's father, had a low forehead and a self-satisfied expression; his uniform sat like a sack on his bulky plebeian figure; on his breast was a medal and a Red Cross Badge. There was little sign of culture, and the luxury was senseless and haphazard, and was as ill fitting as that uniform. The floors irritated him with their brilliant polish, the lustres on the chandelier irritated him, and he was reminded for some reason of the story of the merchant who used to go to the baths with a medal on his neck.

He heard a whispering in the entry; some one was softly snoring. And suddenly from outside came harsh, abrupt, metallic sounds, such as Korolyov had never heard before, and which he did not understand now; they roused strange, unpleasant echoes in his soul.

"I believe nothing would induce me to remain here to live . . ." he thought, and went back to the music-books again.

"Doctor, please come to supper!" the governess called him in a low voice.

He went into supper. The table was large and laid with a vast number of dishes and wines, but there were only two to supper: himself and Christina Dmitryevna. She drank Madeira, ate rapidly, and talked, looking at him through her pince-nez:

"Our workpeople are very contented. We have performances at the factory every winter; the workpeople act themselves. They have lectures with a magic lantern, a splendid tea-room, and everything they want. They are very much attached to us, and when they heard that Lizanka was worse they had a service sung for her. Though they have no education, they have their feelings, too."

"It looks as though you have no man in the house at all," said Korolyov.

"Not one. Pyotr Nikanoritch died a year and a half ago, and left us alone. And so there are the three of us. In the summer we live here, and in winter we live in Moscow, in Polianka. I have been living with them for eleven years — as one of the family."

At supper they served sterlet, chicken rissoles, and stewed fruit; the wines were expensive French wines.

"Please don't stand on ceremony, doctor," said Christina Dmitryevna, eating and wiping her mouth with her fist, and it was evident she found her life here exceedingly pleasant. "Please have some more."

After supper the doctor was shown to his room, where a bed had been made up for him, but he did not feel sleepy. The room was stuffy and it smelt of paint; he put on his coat and went out.

It was cool in the open air; there was already a glimmer of dawn, and all the five blocks of buildings, with their tall chimneys, barracks, and warehouses, were distinctly outlined against the damp air. As it was a holiday, they were not working, and the windows were dark, and in only one of the buildings was there a furnace burning; two windows were crimson, and fire mixed with smoke came from time to time from the chimney. Far away beyond the yard the frogs were croaking and the nightingales singing.

Looking at the factory buildings and the barracks, where the workpeople were asleep, he thought again what he always thought when he saw a factory. They may have performances for the workpeople, magic lanterns, factory doctors, and improvements of all sorts, but, all the same, the workpeople he had met that day on his way from the station did not look in any way different from those he had known long ago in his childhood, before there were factory performances and improvements. As a doctor accustomed to judging correctly of chronic complaints, the radical cause of which was incomprehensible and incurable, he looked upon factories as something baffling, the cause of which also was obscure and not removable, and all the improvements in the life of the factory hands he looked upon not as superfluous, but as comparable with the treatment of incurable illnesses.

"There is something baffling in it, of course . . ." he thought, looking at the crimson windows. "Fifteen hundred or two thousand workpeople are working without rest in unhealthy surroundings, making bad cotton goods, living on the verge of starvation, and only waking from this nightmare at rare intervals in the tavern; a hundred people act as overseers, and the whole life of that hundred is spent in imposing fines, in abuse, in injustice, and only two or three so-called owners enjoy the profits, though they don't work at all, and despise the wretched cotton. But what are the profits, and how do they enjoy them? Madame Lyalikov and her daughter are unhappy—it makes one wretched to look at them; the only one who enjoys her life is Christina Dmitryevna, a stupid, middle-aged maiden lady in pince-nez. And so it appears that all these five blocks of buildings are at work, and inferior cotton is sold in the Eastern markets, simply that Christina Dmitryevna may eat sterlet and drink Madeira."

Suddenly there came a strange noise, the same sound Korolyov had heard before supper. Some one was striking on a sheet of metal near one of the buildings; he struck a note, and then at once checked the vibrations, so that short, abrupt, discordant sounds were produced, rather like "Dair . . . dair . . . dair. . . ." Then there was half a minute of stillness, and from another building there came sounds equally abrupt and unpleasant, lower bass notes: "Drin . . . drin . . . drin. . ." Eleven times. Evidently it was the watchman striking the hour. Near the third building he heard: "Zhuk . . . zhuk . . . zhuk. . . ." And so near all the buildings, and then behind the barracks and beyond the gates. And in the stillness of the night it seemed as though these sounds were uttered by a monster with crimson eyes— the devil himself, who controlled the owners and the work-people alike, and was deceiving both.

Korolyov went out of the yard into the open country.

"Who goes there?" some one called to him at the gates in an abrupt voice.

"It's just like being in prison," he thought, and made no answer.

Here the nightingales and the frogs could be heard more distinctly, and one could feel it was a night in May. From the station came the noise of a train; somewhere in the distance drowsy cocks were crowing; but, all the same, the night was still, the world was sleeping tranquilly. In a field not far from the factory there could be seen the framework of a house and heaps of building material:

Korolyov sat down on the planks and went on thinking.

"The only person who feels happy here is the governess, and the factory hands are working for her gratification. But that's only apparent: she is only the figurehead. The real person, for whom everything is being done, is the devil."

And he thought about the devil, in whom he did not believe, and he looked round at the two windows where the fires were gleaming. It seemed to him that out of those crimson eyes the devil himself was looking at him—that unknown force that had created the mutual relation of the strong and the weak, that coarse blunder which one could never correct. The strong must hinder the weak from living—such was the law of Nature; but only in a newspaper article or in a school book was that intelligible and easily accepted. In the hotchpotch which was everyday life, in the tangle of trivialities out of which human relations were woven, it was no longer a law, but a logical absurdity, when the strong and the weak were both equally victims of their mutual relations, unwillingly submitting to some directing force, unknown, standing outside life, apart from man.

So thought Korolyov, sitting on the planks, and little by little he was possessed by a feeling that this unknown and mysterious force was really close by and looking at him. Meanwhile the east was growing paler, time passed rapidly; when there was not a soul anywhere near, as though everything were dead, the five buildings and their chimneys against the grey background of the dawn had a peculiar look—not the same as by day; one forgot altogether that inside there were steam motors, electricity, telephones, and kept thinking of lake-dwellings, of the Stone Age, feeling the presence of a crude, unconscious force. . . .

And again there came the sound: "Dair . . . dair . . . dair . . . dair . . ." twelve times. Then there was stillness, stillness for half a minute, and at the other end of the yard there rang out.

"Drin . . . drin . . . drin. . . ."

"Horribly disagreeable," thought Korolyov.

"Zhuk . . . zhuk . . ." there resounded from a third place, abruptly, sharply, as though with annoyance—"Zhuk . . . zhuk. . . ."

And it took four minutes to strike twelve. Then there was a hush; and again it seemed as though everything were dead.

Korolyov sat a little longer, then went to the house, but sat up for a good while longer. In the adjoining rooms there was whispering, there was a sound of shuffling slippers and bare feet.

"Is she having another attack?" thought Korolyov.

He went out to have a look at the patient. By now it was quite light in the rooms, and a faint glimmer of sunlight, piercing through the morning mist, quivered on the floor and on the wall of the drawing-room. The door of Liza's room was open, and she was sitting in a low chair beside her bed, with her hair down, wearing a dressing-gown and wrapped in a shawl. The blinds were down on the windows.

"How do you feel?" asked Korolyov.

"Well, thank you."

He touched her pulse, then straightened her hair, that had fallen over her forehead.

"You are not asleep," he said. "It's beautiful weather outside. It's spring. The nightingales are singing, and you sit in the dark and think of something."

She listened and looked into his face; her eyes were sorrowful and intelligent, and it was evident she wanted to say something to him.

"Does this happen to you often?" he said.

She moved her lips, and answered:

"Often, I feel wretched almost every night."

At that moment the watchman in the yard began striking two o'clock. They heard: "Dair . . . dair . . ." and she shuddered.

"Do those knockings worry you?" he asked.

"I don't know. Everything here worries me," she answered, and pondered. "Everything worries me. I hear sympathy in your voice; it seemed to me as soon as I saw you that I could tell you all about it."

"Tell me, I beg you."

"I want to tell you of my opinion. It seems to me that I have no illness, but that I am weary and frightened, because it is bound to be so and cannot be otherwise. Even the healthiest person can't help being uneasy if, for instance, a robber is moving about under his window. I am constantly being doctored," she went on, looking at her knees, and she gave a shy smile. "I am very grateful, of course, and I do not deny that the treatment is a benefit; but I should like to talk, not with a doctor, but with some intimate friend who would understand me and would convince me that I was right or wrong."

"Have you no friends?" asked Korolyov.

"I am lonely. I have a mother; I love her, but, all the same, I am lonely. That's how it happens to be. . . . Lonely people read a great deal, but say little and hear little. Life for them is mysterious; they are mystics and often see the devil where he is not. Lermontov's Tamara was lonely and she saw the devil."

"Do you read a great deal?"

"Yes. You see, my whole time is free from morning till night. I read by day, and by night my head is empty; instead of thoughts there are shadows in it."

"Do you see anything at night?" asked Korolyov.

"No, but I feel. . . ."

She smiled again, raised her eyes to the doctor, and looked at him so sorrowfully, so intelligently; and it seemed to him that she trusted him, and that she wanted to speak frankly to him, and that she thought the same as he did. But she was silent, perhaps waiting for him to speak.

And he knew what to say to her. It was clear to him that she needed as quickly as possible to give up the five buildings and the million if she had it—to leave that devil that looked out at night; it was clear to him, too, that she thought so herself, and was only waiting for some one she trusted to confirm her.

But he did not know how to say it. How? One is shy of asking men under sentence what they have been sentenced for; and in the same way it is awkward to ask very rich people what they want so much money for, why they make such a poor use of their wealth, why they don't give it up, even when they see in it their unhappiness; and if they begin a conversation about it themselves, it is usually embarrassing, awkward, and long.

"How is one to say it?" Korolyov wondered. "And is it necessary to speak?"

And he said what he meant in a roundabout way:

"You in the position of a factory owner and a wealthy heiress are dissatisfied; you don't believe in your right to it; and here now you can't sleep. That, of course, is better than if you were satisfied, slept soundly, and thought everything was satisfactory. Your sleeplessness does you credit; in any case, it is a good sign. In reality, such a conversation as this between us now would have been unthinkable for our parents. At night they did not talk, but slept sound; we, our generation, sleep badly, are restless, but talk a great deal, and are always trying to settle whether we are right or not. For our children or grandchildren that question — whether they are right or not — will have been settled. Things will be clearer for them than for us. Life will be good in fifty years' time; it's only a pity we shall not last out till then. It would be interesting to have a peep at it."

"What will our children and grandchildren do?" asked Liza.

"I don't know. . . . I suppose they will throw it all up and go away."

"Go where?"

"Where? . . . Why, where they like," said Korolyov; and he laughed. "There are lots of places a good, intelligent person can go to."

He glanced at his watch.

"The sun has risen, though," he said. "It is time you were asleep. Undress and sleep soundly. Very glad to have made your acquaintance," he went on, pressing her hand. "You are a good, interesting woman. Good-night!"

He went to his room and went to bed.

In the morning when the carriage was brought round they all came out on to the steps to see him off. Liza, pale and exhausted, was in a white dress as though for a holiday, with a flower in her hair; she looked at him, as yesterday, sorrowfully and intelligently, smiled and talked, and all with an expression as though she wanted to tell him something special, important—him alone. They could hear the larks trilling and the church bells pealing. The windows in the factory buildings were sparkling gaily, and, driving across the yard and afterwards along the road to the station, Korolyov thought neither of the workpeople nor of lake dwellings, nor of the devil, but thought of the time, perhaps close at hand, when life would be as bright and joyous as that still Sunday morning; and he thought how pleasant it was on such a morning in the spring to drive with three horses in a good carriage, and to bask in the sunshine.

A Blight On Society

Marie Sheppard Williams

I

Vickie and Grange.

Victorine and Grangeford de los Alamos.

You don't believe those names, right? Already you think I am

making this up?

Well, you wouldn't have believed those people either.

Vickie and Grangeford were ... sweethearts ...

Yes. That's just what they were.

And listen: don't laugh. If you laugh, I'll—I'll rip your nose off, that's what I'll do.

I'm the only one who gets to laugh.

II

As part of my job at the agency I do intake, among other things.

Brenda Pauley, who is a rehab counselor at the state agency—our referring agency—called me one day.

I've got one for you: her sardonic, flat, pained voice came over the telephone. Brenda is probably my favorite counselor over there: she never bullshits me, she shoots absolutely straight, her attitudes are almost a hundred percent negative, I find her very funny.

I've got a woman named Victorine de los Alamos, she said that day. Listen, you'll like her, she said: she's diabetic, she's got some vision left, a lot of other problems, and get this, her husband also became diabetic recently and is starting to lose vision too.

Are they both on Disability? I asked.

The Social Security fund disability section: that's what I was talking about.

Not yet, said Brenda. They will be in a couple of months. Or at least Vickie will. Right now they're on SSI.

SSI is Supplemental Security Income, in case you don't know it. A kind of welfare.

I wouldn't want to shit you, said Brenda: I'm probably the only professional in town who likes them. Vickie's doctor hates them, and their social worker hates them, Legal Aid hates them, Methodist Hospital hates them, listen, their garbage collector probably hates them, the mailman probably hates them.

I laughed. I know Brenda. I think I do. Why's that, Bren? I said.

Well, you know, she said. They're a multiproblem couple. A blight on society. The sty in the eye of the nation, you should excuse the expression. They've got every agency in town involved in their case. And the thing is, they're not a bit ashamed or depressed or anything. They're making a very good life out of it.

Multiproblem: you have to understand that this was right at the height of the great Multiproblem Discovery. Would you believe it, social workers and such had worked for years with people and until the time of the Great Discovery they had assumed that every one of those people had only one problem each. The notion that some of them had two or more at the same time: say, poverty and handicap and disease and illiteracy: that notion was an absolute mindblower to professionals. And didn't they love the multiproblem families at first? Oh, they did, for a while; well, they had a category for them, you see. If they put them into the category, they could understand them. This love did not however last: it soon became apparent that even if you knew what to call them, you still couldn't do anything about them. Social workers hate things they can't do anything about.

Well, if you like them, I'll like them, I said to Brenda. Probably. I like them, Brenda says. But you know me, I'm very strange.

Brenda brings them in to talk to me. Vickie—I see on the referral information that B. has handed to me—is fifty-five years old. She is gray haired and quiet. Grange is fifty-four, and awful. (The referral information does not say that, I am just throwing that in for you.) Grange sits hunched forward in one of the chairs in front of my desk: heavyset, florid, mustached, big calculating smile flashing on and off as he psychs me out. Oh, I've seen his kind: I am onto him. He clutches a battered tweed hat in both hands in his lap.

Hello, hello, he says. I'm really glad to meet you. Brenda here, Brenda says you know your onions, and what Brenda says goes a long way with me …

Hello, Grange, I say. I'm glad to meet you. And Vickie, how are you?

She's fine today, Grange says. She's really pretty good today.

He takes one hand off the tweed hat and reaches for his wife's hand, squeezes it. He turns to her: You're fine, aren't you Vickie? Vickie smiles then; a singularly sweet and piercing smile that reaches out to meet him. I touch Vickie's shoulder: How about if Vickie tells me? I say.

Grange: Oh, Vickie doesn't talk much. She won't tell you how she really is. She'll say she's just fine. I'm the talker here.

Me: Yes, well, I'd really like to get to know Vickie a little. I'd really like to hear it from Vickie.

Grange: Now that makes sense. That makes a lot of sense.

Talk, Vickie.

Oh, Grange is the talker, says Vickie softly. Grange usually talks for me.

Grange gives me his flashing, apologetic, and cringing smile again: that is also merry and impudent. What did I tell you? he says.

I'm kind of shy, murmurs Vickie.

That's all right, Vickie, Grange says. He holds her hand. She smiles at him, that piercing bright smile again: he smiles back at her. We're very devoted to each other, he says. We're very devoted. Two tears squeeze out of his eyes and straggle down the sides of his nose, past his grin.

And now she's blind, he says; and two more tears roll down.

God. He looks like a big sincere crocodile. Smiling. Of course I like him, how could I not like him, he is so awful? I look at Brenda as they all get up to go, bundle back into their coats. And Bren looks at me as they leave, her face twisted and sardonic: how about that? the look says. I knew you'd like them. You're as strange as I am. The look says.

I'm going out with Tommy Rizzio these days, Brenda says to me as we walk down the stairs toward the front door of the agency. Had you heard? Tommy Rizzio! I say. No. I hadn't heard. Jesus, Brenda, you've got to be kidding, I think to myself. Tommy Rizzio. Not a good idea. In my opinion.

III

I saw a lot of Vickie after that, when she came to our agency as a student. At the agency, they teach people how to cope with being blind. I saw her when specific problems came up, or when she just wanted someone to talk to—after a while she did begin to talk—or when I met her by accident in the hallway. She talked about death and Grange. She was afraid to die and she loved Grange.

Afraid To Die I could get my teeth into. Talk to me about it, I told her. Talk to me about death, what does it mean to you to die, Vickie? (What Does That Mean To You—that is a professional phrase, like Mmm-hmm. They teach it to all of us. Actually, I don't mean to make fun of it; it comes in very useful at times; and it reflects a useful idea, that people say things in a way to hide from themselves the real meaning; and that the words lie unless you squeeze the truth out of them.) Bur Vickie couldn't talk about death. She could only say that she had a great fear, was very afraid. But then she would mention Grange, and the marvelous smile would come, and death would be forgotten for that day.

I was sixteen when I met him, she tells me. He was fifteen. She says that they were married in three months and have been together ever since; she says they have lived in many places, California, Wisconsin, Michigan, trying one venture and another. She says they have never had a real house until now; now they live in a house across the river in St. Paul, and this is wonderful to them.

One day Vickie didn't come to school. I called and talked to Grange and didn't get anything very satisfactory out of him. Victorine's foot was bothering her, he said. And the doctors were really screwing them over, the doctors didn't know what they were doing. He bitched and cried and laughed over the telephone. But he said Vickie would come back to school in a few days.

She didn't come back.

Brenda called me. Look, she said, Grange won't let me talk to Vickie; I'm going out there to find out for myself what's going on.

I asked her if I could go along. Sure, she said. Asking is a necessary formality; the form is that the client always and forever belongs to the referring counselor. Even in Bren's case, I felt that it was as well to stick to the ceremony.

IV

So the next day we drive up to the house in Brenda's car. The house is a neat white rambler affair, with an attached garage. The garage door has an American flag painted on it. Big: it covers the whole door.

Will you look at that, I say to Brenda. Far out, she says.

Do they rent? I say.

Oh, sure, says Bren.

They never owned anything in their lives, says Bren. Must be a very tolerant land-lord, I say.

We go in. The living room is paneled in mirrored squares that reflect furniture and plants to infinity. Even the ceiling is mirrored. In front of the mirrored fire-place and reflected in it is—Guess. You can't guess? No, not in a million years—a life-size plaster statue of Jesus Christ, painted in bright colors.

My goodness, says Brenda: this is a remarkable room.

Do you like it, says Grange. I did it. I thought of it. I put the mirrors up. I painted the statue.

It's, ah, wonderful, says Brenda. You're very talented, Grange. (That's another thing they teach us in school: Perjury. There's a course in it. I swear to god.)

Oh I love to paint things, Grange says. Of Course I bought the statue, but the painting is mine. Do you like it?

Oh yes, we say. I got an A+ in Perjury. I believe Brenda did too.

Look, I'll show you another one, Grange says. He leads us over to a corner of the mirrored room. On a table is a painted statue about eighteen inches high, this one of two people, a man and a woman, embracing naked, looking into one another's eyes.

It's Adam and Eve, Grange says. His uncertain smile flickers on and off.

Adam and Eve! we exclaim. Goodness.

Grange lowers his voice to a confidential mutter. There's something special about them, he says. Do you notice anything special about them?

We look. Don't see anything. Grange tips us off: kindly.

Notice Adam's mustache, he says.

Adam has a painted mustache. Notice Eve's hair.

Eve's hair is painted gray.

Brenda gets it before I do.

It's you and Vickie, isn't it? she says.

Yes it is, Grange says, his hands clasped in front of him, gazing at the statue. It's me and Vickie. I had to have my little secret there didn't I? It just came to me, what I would do ...

Well—God. What can you say?

I say: It's marvelous, Grange. It's a great idea. It's a wonderful idea. You're a wonderful artist, Grange.

He smiles at me, a big smile full of teeth. Yes I am, he says: pretty good. If I say so myself.

Lord. I am afraid to look at Brenda. I know I'll laugh. I am very touched by the statue but I know I'll laugh anyway. If I look at her. You see, it is in me to laugh at things: life, death, comedy, tragedy, all of it. It is in me to laugh. It is the way I save myself. Do you have a way to save yourself? What is your way? I am really interested in your answer.

V

Grange showed us into the bedroom where Vickie was waiting for us, and then he left us alone with her. Vickie was in bed, lying against heaped-up pillows in a canopy bed. The canopy was made of purple crepe paper: pleated and looped and shirred and scalloped. And set off—set off? my god: it needed to be set off?—with strips of gold rickrack tacked onto it with goldheaded thumbtacks. The devil of laughter in me began to jump up and down and to choke.

I let Brenda take the lead: What an interesting bed, Vickie, she said.

It's pretty, isn't it, said Vickie. Grange thought of it and I helped him do it. Before, you know.

Before you lost vision, Vickie? said Brenda. Yes, Vickie said. Before.

What's happening with you now, Vickie, said Brenda. Oh, it's my foot, said Vickie. My toe.

Well what's wrong with your toe?

Oh, well, it had a blister on it and then it got worse and the doctor said I should keep off of it or it might turn into gangrene and I did keep off it but now it's gangrene anyway I think ... Vickie began to cry.

Gangrene. I looked at her, lying on the heaped pillows in the purple crepe-paper bed, a gray-haired, faded, strong-looking middle-aged woman. Who had gangrene.

Who lived in a house of mirrors, whose husband painted her as Eve on a plaster statue.

Oh, you know, the laughing devil in me loved it, the devil went mad. Purple crepe-paper bed canopy, he pointed out, and gangrene! Too much. Too much.

This was the point at which I could have hoped that Brenda would take over—after all, Vickie was her client. But Brenda dropped out on me. She sat in a bentwood rocker by the window and the sun streamed in past white starched ruffled cotton curtains and lighted her: a smart and attractive woman, thirty or so, blonde short hair exquisitely cut, beautiful restrained figure in tasteful clothes, and unwilling apparently to say the next thing.

(I will never have Brenda's style. I try; god knows I do try; but I always end up looking like a refugee from a garage sale. "Funky," people say. They also say—the nicest ones, the ones who actually like me, and not everybody does—the ones who like me say that I have my own style. I take some consolation from this idea.)

So it was up to me. God—was this fair? I was the one who saw everything so goddamn funny: what could I say?

Oh, well, I did know what I had to say. It did come to me: things do. In the clutch, things do come. That's where the training figures in.

Is it death, Vickie, I asked. Is it that you think you will die of this?

She nodded a little and the tears came faster and became shaking sobs.

I sat down next to her on the bed, I took her in my arms and held her and smoothed her gray hair.

Cry, Vickie, I said. It won't be all right, this is not going to be all right, I won't tell you that, but you can cry anyway, and maybe that will help some ...

I looked over at Brenda, who was still sitting in the bentwood rocker. I motioned to her. She got up and came to the other side of the bed and sat on it and held Vickie from that side. So there we were, two fortunate cynical women, holding a sobbing Vickie with her gangrenous toe under the purple crepe-paper canopy.

VI

Brenda and I are both divorced. It is a bond between us: one of many. We both married the kind of man that fortunate cynical intelligent women often do seem to marry in this society nowadays. They even write books about us: *Smart Women, Foolish Choices.* Titles like that. Each of us has a daughter, Brenda and me, I mean. Brenda's daughter is eight years old. My daughter was eight when the divorce occurred.

Why, Mama, my daughter pleaded on the day of the divorce.

Why did you do it?

We don't love each other anymore, Margaret, I said. I don't love your Daddy any more. He doesn't love me. We just can't live together ....

It's not true! she said. It's not true.

It is true, Margaret, I said.

But the thing is, if I couldn't live with Bud, who the hell could I live with? Nobody? Maybe nobody. Maybe I just don't have it in me.

Margaret plotted for years to get me and Bud back together. Her plots were sinister and extraordinary. I watched her with amazement: that she was capable of such calculation, manipulation.

She also plotted and planned to keep other men out of my life. In this plotting she was more successful.

One night at two a.m. I was in a clinch in the living room with a guy named Jason O'Fallon. I don't suppose I loved him, but I did like him, in a way: he amused me: and he touched me: he was so sad and crazy. Margaret came down the stairs in her new Christmas robe and snapped on the overhead light. O'Fallon and I jerked out of our embrace and stared at her: she was beautiful, thirteen years old, standing on the stairs. She accused us with enormous brown eyes: What exactly, she said, staring over me at O'Fallon, are your intentions toward my mother?

I couldn't help it, I laughed. And I gave her an answer.

Margaret, I said, O'Fallon wants to screw me and I want to save O'Fallon's soul.

Well, O'Fallon was horrified: my god, he said. Good Christ.

And that was pretty much the end of that romance. There was an occasional phone call or drop-in visit after that; but basically it was finished. Well, you see, she made me see him funny.

When she graduated from high school—she was living with her father in Santa Monica at the time—I went out there for the ceremony. As the three of us walked on the Santa Monica pier after the graduation, Margaret came between Bud and me and put an arm around each of us.

She sighed—ahhh-h-h-h: and I knew something awful was coming. The white carnation that the headmaster had given her as he sent her forth into the world dangled delicate from the fingers of the hand that she rested on my waist. This, she said, smiled, sighed on the warm summer night air: this is the realization of a brokenhearted eight-year-old's dream ...

Yes, honest to god, she really said that.

Oh, Margaret, for god's sake, I said.

No, it really is, she said. You believe it, don't you Daddy?

Bud smiled at her in hopeless infatuation. My beautiful, beautiful daughter: he said.

See, the thing is, I did him some harm too, in my quest for, what do they call it, Self. Maybe we could have worked it out. I wonder if we could have worked it out.

No. Never. That was not an answer. What is an answer? I don't know. There are questions' that have no answers. Maybe this is a question with no answer.

VII

As I hold Vickie, sobbing, in my arms, I am thinking of: Bud, Margaret, the mirrors, the Jesus statue, O'Fallon, Brenda's ex-husband whom I never knew. He was a bastard: that was all she ever told me about him. I don't know, Brenda was probably not all that easy either. None of us are, these days. You know us: the cynical strong intelligent talented women, fighting tooth and fucking nail for our rights.

I held Vickie and rocked her and murmured words to her, and Brenda held her and was silent. After a while:

Talk to us about it, Vickie, I said.

It's, it's, they might have to cut my toe off, she said, snuffling. You've been so brave about it all up to now, Vickie, I said.

Why now? This?

This is the way it starts, she said. With one toe. Then they cut off your foot.

That might happen, yes, I said.

You die then, said Vickie. They cut off more and more, and pretty soon there's no more to cut off, and then you die ...

Is it pain that you're afraid of, Vickie? I said.

No, said Vickie. Not pain.

Is it what happens to you after you die that scares you so, Vickie?

No, no, that's all right, God takes me home, I'm not afraid of that ... She trembled and sobbed in my arms.

What then, Vickie?

Oh, she said, oh, it's that I have to go alone. It's that Grange can't come with me ... I have to leave Grange alone ...

So that's it. So that's it. Something so far outside of my understanding that I feel my mind stretching into a whole new shape to get it in: the sentimental idea of love. The real for Christ's sake thing. Love. In a middle-aged gray-haired woman with a gangrenous toe under a purple crepe-paper canopy made for her by a fat and tasteless grinning oaf. On Welfare.

Oh, my devil who saves me is laughing to split his sides: can you hear him? Surely his laughter is so loud that you can hear it.

(Saves me?)

VIII

Grange walked us out to Brenda's car. The red-white-blue garage door dazzled in the sun.

Thank you for coming, he said. It means a lot to Vickie that you came.

Thanks for letting us come, said Brenda. Think nothing of it, he said.

Your garage door is spectacular, Grange, I said. Did you paint it? Oh! Yes! he said. I change it for every holiday, he said.

Every holiday? I said.

Every single one, he said. And sometimes I put in one for a holiday no one would ordinarily think of, the summer solstice for example. If I happen to want to. Vickie's birthday.

It's a marvelous idea, I said.

Yes, isn't it? he said. Isn't it marvelous? Isn't it just marvelous?

IX

So we drove home, Brenda and I. We were quiet for a while. She drove along the freeway back toward the agency. The traffic got heavier.

Then: Christmas, I said. A big red Santa. Plus a nativity scene.

And listen, Halloween. A big orange pumpkin.

Ghosts! Skeletons!

We started to laugh. Washington's birthday! Cascades of laughter. Thanksgiving! A Thanksgiving turkey! Arbor Day! Trees! On the, on the garage! And listen, gallons and gallons of paint! The taxpayers are buying gallons of paint for this project! Oh if they only knew, god if they only knew ... listen, Valentine's Day ...

God. It's a wonder we didn't hit another car. Out there on the freeway.

It's a wonder we didn't get killed.

Valentine's Day.

X

We don't talk about it very often, Brenda and I. Once in a while. But it is there connecting us: we have an important connecting memory.

Brenda brings me news of them sometimes.

Grange and Vickie have moved to Wisconsin, she says. Vickie is going to a rehab center there. The state counselor called me to ask for our records ...

One day: Vickie's had her foot amputated.

And another day: Vickie died, Brenda says. Grange called me.

How did he sound? I say.

Like always, she says. Full of, you know, life ... I mean, sad, but kind of energetic ...

I wonder what will become of him, I say.

I wonder, she says.

Last week, I met Brenda for lunch. She is in the process of getting her second divorce: from Tommy Rizzio, who turned out to be a bastard too.

I told her that I was going to write a story about Vickie and Grange.

Will you let me read it? she said.

Yes, I'll let you read it, I said. Sure.

Maybe I will. Maybe I won't.

I don't know, I am a taxpayer too, and I feel that my money was well spent in that case. And, thinking about it, suddenly I see myself rushing forward to embrace my death, my only lover: my promised end, my goal, surcease. Lord, sometimes I feel like a member of the poor: I feel like I need to be on some special kind of Welfare.

SECTION 3
Calamities

La malattia dice chi siamo
Illnesses tell us what we are

Italian Proverb

The Sick Child

Henook-Makhewe-Kelenaka (Angel de Cora)

It was about sunset when I, a little child, was sent with a handful of powdered tobacco leaves and red feathers to make an offering to the spirit who had caused the sickness of my little sister. It had been a long, hard winter, and the snow lay deep on the prairie as far as the eye could reach. The medicine-woman's directions had been that the offering must be laid upon the naked earth, and that to find it I must face toward the setting sun.

I was taught the prayer: "Spirit grandfather, I offer this to thee. I pray thee restore my little sister to health." Full of reverence and a strong faith that I could appease the anger of the spirit, I started out to plead for the life of our little one.

But now where was a spot of earth to be found in all that white monotony? They had talked of death at the house. I hoped that my little sister would live, but I was afraid of nature.

I reached a little spring. I looked down to its pebbly bottom, wondering whether I should leave my offering there, or keep on in search of a spot of earth. If I put my offering in the water, would it reach the bottom and touch the earth, or would it float away, as it had always done when I made my offering to the water spirit?

Once more I started on in my search of the bare ground.

The surface was crusted in some places, and walking was easy; in other places I would wade through a foot or more of snow. Often I paused, thinking to clear the snow away in some place and there lay my offering. But no, my faith must be in nature, and I must trust to it to lay bare the earth.

It was a hard struggle for so small a child.

I went on and on; the reeds were waving their tasselled ends in the wind. I stopped and looked at them. A reed, whirling in the wind, had formed a space round its stem, making a loose socket. I stood looking into the opening. The reed must be rooted in the ground, and the hole must follow the stem to the earth. If I poured my offerings into the hole, surely they must reach the ground; so I said the prayer I had been taught, and dropped my tobacco and red feathers into the opening that nature itself had created.

No sooner was the sacrifice accomplished than a feeling of doubt and fear thrilled me. What if my offering should never reach the earth? Would my little sister die?

Not till I turned homeward did I realize how cold I was. When at last I reached the house they took me in and warmed me, but did not question me, and I said nothing. Every one was sad, for the little one had grown worse.

The next day the medicine woman said my little sister was beyond hope; she could not live. Then bitter remorse was mine, for I thought I had been unfaithful, and therefore my little sister was to be called to the spirit-land. I was a silent child, and did not utter my feelings; my remorse was intense.

My parents would not listen to what the medicine-woman had said, but clung to hope. As soon as she had gone, they sent for a medicine-man who lived many miles away.

He arrived about dark. He was a large man, with a sad, gentle face. His presence had always filled me with awe, and that night it was especially so, for he was coming as a holy man. He entered the room where the baby lay, and took a seat, hardly noticing any one. There was silence saving only for the tinkling of the little tin ornaments on his medicine-bag. He began to speak: "A soul has departed from this house, gone to the spirit-land. As I came I saw luminous vapor above the house. It ascended, it grew less, it was gone on its way to the spirit-land. It was the spirit of the little child who is sick; she still breathes, but her spirit is beyond our reach. If medicine will ease her pain, I will do what I can."

He stood up and blessed the four corners of the earth with song. Then, according to the usual custom of medicine-doctors, he began reciting the vision that had given him the right to be a medicine-man. The ruling force of the vision had been in the form of a bear. To it he addressed his prayer, saying: "Inasmuch as thou hast given me power to cure the sick, and in one case allowing me to unite spirit and body again, if thou seest fit, allow me to recall the spirit of this child to its body once more." He asked that the coverings be taken off the baby, and that it be brought into the middle of the room. Then, as he sang, he danced slowly around the little form. When the song was finished, he blessed the child, and then prepared the medicine, stirring into water some ground herbs. This he took into his mouth and sprinkled it over the little body. Another mixture he gave her to drink.

Almost instantly there was a change; the little one began to breathe more easily, and as the night wore on she seemed to suffer less. Finally she opened her eyes, looked into mother's face, and smiled. The medicine-man, seeing it, said that the end was near, and though he gave her more medicine, the spirit, he said, would never return.

After saying words of comfort, he took his departure, refusing to take a pony and some blankets that were offered him, saying that he had been unable to hold the spirit back, and had no right to accept the gifts.

The next morning I found the room all cleared away, and my mother sat sewing on a little white gown. The bright red trimming caught my eye. I came to her and asked, "Please mother, tell me for whom is that, and why do you make it so pretty?" She made no answer, but bent over her work. I leaned forward that I might look into her face and repeat my question. I bent down, and, oh! the tears were falling fast down her cheeks. Then we were told that our little sister was gone to the spirit-land, and we must not talk about her. We felt of her and kissed her, but she made no response. Then I realized what death meant. Remorse again seized me, but I was silent.

Mrs. Cassidy's Last Year

Mary Gordon

Mr. Cassidy knew he couldn't go to Communion. He had sinned against charity. He had wanted his wife dead.

The intention had been his, and the desire. She would not go back to bed. She had lifted the table that held her breakfast (it was unfair, it was unfair to all of them, that the old woman should be so strong and so immobile). She had lifted the table above her head and sent it crashing to the floor in front of him.

"Rose," he had said, bending, wondering how he would get scrambled egg, coffee, cranberry juice (which she had said she liked, the color of it) out of the garden pattern on the carpet. That was the sort of thing she knew but would not tell him now. She would laugh, wicked and bland-faced as an egg, when he did the wrong thing. But never say what was right, although she knew it, and her tongue was not dead for curses, for reports of crimes.

"Shithawk," she would shout at him horn her bedroom. "Bastard son of a whore." Or more mildly, "Pimp," or "Fathead fart."

Old words, curses heard from soldiers on the boat or somebody's street children. Never spoken by her until now. Punishing him, though he had kept his promise.

He was trying to pick up the scrambled eggs with a paper napkin. The napkin broke, then shredded when he tried to squeeze the egg into what was left of it. He was on his knees on the carpet, scraping egg, white shreds of paper, purple fuzz from the trees in the carpet.

"Shitscraper," she laughed at him on his knees.

And then he wished in his heart most purely for the woman to be dead.

The doorbell rang. His son and his son's wife. Shame that they should see him so, kneeling, bearing curses, cursing in his heart.

"Pa," said Toni, kneeling next to him. "You see what we mean."

"She's too much for you," said Mr. Cassidy's son Tom. Self-made man, thought Mr. Cassidy. Good time Charlie. Every joke a punchline like a whip.

No one would say his wife was too much for him.

"Swear," she had said, lying next to him in bed when they were each no more than thirty. Her eyes were wild then. What had made her think of it? No sickness near them, and fearful age some continent like Africa, with no one they knew well. What had put the thought to her, and the wildness, so that her nails bit into his palm, as if she knew small pain would preserve his memory.

"Swear you will let me die in my own bed. Swear you won't let them take me away."

He swore, her nails making dents in his palms, a dull shallow pain, not sharp, blue-green or purplish.

He had sworn.

On his knees now beside his daughter-in-law, his son.

"She is not too much for me. She is my wife."

"Leave him then, Toni," said Tom. "Let him do it himself if it's so goddamn easy. Serve him right. Let him learn the hard way. He couldn't do it if he didn't have us, the slobs around the corner."

Years of hatred now come out, punishing for not being loved best, of the family's children not most prized. Nothing is forgiven, thought the old man, rising to his feet, his hand on his daughter-in-law's squarish shoulder.

He knelt before the altar of God. The young priest, bright-haired, faced them, arms open, a good little son.

No sons priests. He thought how he was old enough now to have a priest a grandson. This boy before him, vested and ordained, could have been one of the ones who followed behind holding tools. When there was time. He thought of Tom looking down at his father who knelt trying to pick up food. Tom for whom there had been no time. Families were this: the bulk, the knot of memory, wounds remembered not only because they had set on the soft, the pliable wax of childhood, motherhood, fatherhood, closeness to death. Wounds most deeply set and best remembered because families are days, the sameness of days and words, hammer blows, smothering, breath grabbed, memory on the soft skull, in the lungs, not once only but again and again the same. The words and the starvation.

Tom would not forget, would not forgive him. Children thought themselves the only wounded.

Should we let ourselves in for it, year after year, he asked in prayer, believing God did not hear him.

Tom would not forgive him for being the man he was. A man who paid debts, kept promises. Mr. Cassidy knelt up straighter, proud of himself before God.

Because of the way he had to be. He knelt back again, not proud. As much sense to be proud of the color of his hair. As much choice.

It was his wife who was the proud one. As if she thought it could have been some other way. The house, the children. He knew, being who they were they must have a house like that, children like that. Being who they were to the world. Having their faces.

As if she thought with some wrong turning these things might have been wasted. Herself a slattern, him drunk, them living in a tin shack, children dead or missing.

One was dead. John, the favorite, lost somewhere in a plane. The war dead. There was his name on the plaque near the altar. With the other town boys. And she had never forgiven him. For what he did not know. For helping bring that child into the world? Better, she said, to have borne none than the pain of losing this one, the most beautiful, the bravest. She turned from him then, letting some shelf drop, like a merchant at the hour of closing. And Tom had not forgotten the grief at his brother's death, knowing he could not have closed his mother's heart like that.

Mr. Cassidy saw they were all so unhappy, hated each other so because they thought things could be different. As he had thought of his wife. He had imagined she could be different if she wanted to. Which had angered him. Which was not, was almost never, the truth about things.

Things were as they were going to be, he thought, watching the boy-faced priest giving out Communion. Who were the others not receiving? Teenagers, pimpled, believing themselves in sin. He wanted to tell them they were not. He was sure they were not. Mothers with babies. Not going to Communion because they took the pill, it must be. He thought they should not stay away, although he thought they should not do what they had been told not to. He knew that the others in their seats were there for the heat of their bodies. While he sat back for the cold-ness of his heart, a heart that had wished his wife dead. He had wished the one dead he had promised he would love forever.

The boy priest blessed the congregation. Including Mr. Cassidy himself.

"Pa," said Tom, walking beside his father, opening the car door for him. "You see what we mean about her?"

"It was my fault. I forgot."

"Forgot what?" said Tom, emptying his car ashtray onto the church parking lot. Not my son, thought Mr. Cassidy, turning his head.

"How she is," said Mr. Cassidy. "I lost my temper."

"Pa, you're not God," said Tom. His hands were on the steering wheel, angry. His mother's.

"Okay," said Toni. "But look, Pa, you've been a saint to her. But she's not the woman she was. Not the woman we knew."

"She's the woman I married."

"Not any more," said Toni, wife of her husband.

If not, then who? People were the same. They kept their bodies. They did not become someone else. Rose was the woman he had married, a green girl, high-colored, with beautifully cut nostrils, hair that fell down always, hair she pinned up swiftly, with anger. She had been a housemaid and he a chauffeur. He had taken her to the ocean. They wore straw hats. They were not different people now. She was the girl he had seen first, the woman he had married, the mother of his children, the woman he had promised: Don't let them take me. Let me die in my own bed.

"Supposing it was yourself and Tom, then, Toni," said Mr. Cassidy, remembering himself a gentleman. "What would you want him to do? Would you want him to break his promise?"

"I hope I'd never make him promise anything like that," said Toni.

"But if you did?"

"I don't believe in those kinds of promises."

"My father thinks he's God. You have to understand. There's no two ways about anything."

For what was his son now refusing to forgive him? He was silent now, sitting in the back of the car. He looked at the top of his daughter-in-law's head, blond now, like some kind of circus candy. She had never been blond. Why did they do it? Try to be what they were not born to. Rose did not.

"What I wish you'd get through your head, Pa, is that it's me and Toni carrying the load. I suppose you forget where all the suppers come from?"

"I don't forget."

"Why don't you think of Toni for once?"

"I think of her, Tom, and you too. I know what you do. I'm very grateful. Mom is grateful, too, or she would be."

But first I think of my wife to whom I made vows. And whom I promised.

"The doctor thinks you're nuts, you know that, don't you?" said Tom. "Rafferty thinks you're nuts to try and keep her. He thinks we're nuts to go along with you. He says he washes his hands of the whole bunch of us."

The doctor washes his hands, thought Mr. Cassidy, seeing Leo Rafferty, hale as a dog, at his office sink.

The important thing was not to forget she was the woman he had married.

So he could leave the house, so he could leave her alone, he strapped her into the bed. Her curses were worst when he released her. She had grown a beard this last year, like a goat.

Like a man?

No.

He remembered her as she was when she was first his wife. A white nightgown, then as now. So she was the same. He'd been told it smelled different a virgin's first time. And never that way again. Some blood. Not much. As if she hadn't minded.

He sat her in the chair in front of the television. They had Mass now on television for sick people, people like her. She pushed the button on the little box that could change channels from across the room. One of their grandsons was a TV repairman. He had done it for them when she got sick. She pushed the button to a station that showed cartoons. Mice in capes, cats outraged. Some stories now with colored children. He boiled an egg for her lunch.

She sat chewing, looking at the television. What was that look in her eyes now? Why did he want to call it wickedness? Because it was blank and hateful. Because there was no light. Eyes should have light. There should be something behind them. That was dangerous, nothing behind her eyes but hate. Sullen like a bull kept from a cow. Sex mad. Why did that look make him think of sex? Sometimes he was afraid she wanted it.

He did not know what he would do.

She slept. He slept in the chair across from her.

The clock went off for her medicine. He got up from the chair, gauging the weather. Sometimes the sky was green this time of year. It was warm when it should not be. He didn't like that. The mixup made him shaky. It made him say to himself, "Now I am old."

He brought her the medicine. Three pills, red and grey, red and yellow, dark pink. Two just to keep her quiet. Sometimes she sucked them and spat them out when they melted and she got the bad taste. She thought they were candy. It was their fault for making them those colors. But it was something else he had to think about. He had to make sure she swallowed them right away.

Today she was not going to swallow. He could see that by the way her eyes looked at the television. The way she set her mouth so he could see what she had done with the pills, kept them in a pocket in her cheek, as if for storage.

"Rose," he said, stepping between her and the television, breaking her gaze. "You've got to swallow the pills. They cost money."

She tried to look over his shoulder. On the screen an ostrich, dressed in colored stockings, danced down the road. He could see she was not listening to him. And he tried to remember what the young priest had said when he came to bring Communion, what his daughter June had said. Be patient with her. Humor her. She can't help what she does. She's not the woman she once was.

She is the same.

"Hey, my Rose, won't you just swallow the pills for me. Like my girl."

She pushed him out of the way. So she could go on watching the television. He knelt down next to her.

"Come on, girleen. It's the pills make you better."

She gazed over the top of his head. He stood up, remembering what was done to animals.

He stroked her throat as he had stroked the throats of dogs and horses, a boy on a farm. He stroked the old woman's loose, papery throat, and said, "Swallow, then, just swallow."

She looked over his shoulder at the television. She kept the pills in a corner of her mouth.

It was making him angry. He put one finger above her lip under her nose and one below her chin, so that she would not be able to open her mouth. She breathed through her nose like a patient animal. She went on looking at the television. She did not swallow.

"You swallow them, Rose, this instant," he said, clamping her mouth shut. "They cost money. The doctor says you must. You're throwing good money down the drain."

Now she was watching a lion and a polar bear dancing. There were pianos in their cages.

He knew he must move away or his anger would make him do something. He had promised he would not be angry. He would remember who she was.

He went into the kitchen with a new idea. He would give her something sweet that would make her want to swallow. There was ice cream in the refrigerator. Strawberry that she liked. He removed each strawberry and placed it in the sink so she would not chew and then get the taste of the medicine. And then spit it out, leaving him, leaving them both no better than when they began.

He brought the dish of ice cream to her in the living room. She was sitting staring at the television with her mouth open. Perhaps she had opened her mouth to laugh? At what? At what was this grown woman laughing? A zebra was playing a xylophone while his zebra wife hung striped pajamas on a line.

In opening her mouth, she had let the pills fall together onto her lap. He saw the three of them, wet, stuck together, at the center of her lap. He thought he would take the pills and simply hide them in the ice cream. He bent to fish them from the valley of her lap.

And then she screamed at him. And then she stood up.

He was astonished at her power. She had not stood by herself for seven months. She put one arm in front of her breasts and raised the other against him, knocking him heavily to the floor.

"No," she shouted, her voice younger, stronger, the voice of a well young man. "Don't think you can have it now. That's what you're after. That's what you're always after. You want to get into it. I'm not one of your whores. You always thought it was such a great prize. I wish you'd have it cut off. I'd like to cut it off."

And she walked out of the house. He could see her wandering up and down the street in the darkness.

He dragged himself over to the chair and propped himself against it so he could watch her through the window. But he knew he could not move any farther. His leg was light and foolish underneath him, and burning with pain. He could not move any more, not even to the telephone that was half a yard away from him. He could see her body, visible through her nightgown, as she walked the street in front of the house.

He wondered if he should call out or be silent. He did not know how far she would walk. He could imagine her walking until the land stopped, and then into the water. He could not stop her. He would not raise his voice.

There was that pain in his leg that absorbed him strangely, as if it were the pain of someone else. He knew the leg was broken. "I have broken my leg," he kept saying to himself, trying to connect the words and the burning.

But then he remembered what it meant. He would not be able to walk. He would not be able to take care of her.

"Rose," he shouted, trying to move toward the window.

And then, knowing he could not move and she could not hear him, "Help."

He could see the green numbers on the clock, alive as cat's eyes. He could see his wife walking in the middle of the street. At least she was not walking far. But no one was coming to help her.

He would have to call for help. And he knew what it meant: they would take her away somewhere. No one would take care of her in the house if he did not. And he could not move.

No one could hear him shouting. No one but he could see his wife, wandering up and down the street in her nightgown.

They would take her away. He could see it; he could hear the noises. Policemen in blue, car radios reporting other disasters, young boys writing his words down in notebooks. And doctors, white coats, white shoes, wheeling her out. Her strapped. She would curse him. She would curse him rightly for having broken his promise. And the young men would wheel her out. Almost everyone was younger than he now. And he could hear how she would be as they wheeled her past him, rightly cursing.

Now he could see her weaving in the middle of the street. He heard a car slam on its brakes to avoid her. He thought someone would have to stop then. But he heard the car go on down to the corner.

No one could hear him shouting in the living room. The windows were shut; it was late October. There was a high bulk of grey cloud, showing islands of fierce, acidic blue. He would have to do something to get someone's attention before the sky became utterly dark and the drivers could not see her wandering before their cars. He could see her wandering; he could see the set of her angry back. She was wearing only her nightgown. He would have to get someone to bring her in before she died of cold.

The only objects he could reach were the figurines that covered the low table beside him. He picked one up: a bust of Robert Kennedy. He threw it through the window. The breaking glass made a violent, disgraceful noise. It was the sound of disaster he wanted. It must bring help.

He lay still for ten minutes, waiting, looking at the clock. He could see her walking, cursing. She could not hear him. He was afraid no one could hear him. He picked up another figurine, a bicentennial eagle and threw it through the window next to the one he had just broken. Then he picked up another and threw it through the window next to that. He went on: six windows. He went on until he had broken every window in the front of the house.

He had ruined his house. The one surprising thing of his long lifetime. The broken glass winked like green jewels, hard sea creatures, on the purple carpet. He looked at what he had destroyed. He would never have done it; it was something he would never have done. But he would not have believed he was a man who could not keep his promise.

In the dark he lay and prayed that someone would come and get her. That was the only thing now to pray for; the one thing he had asked God to keep back. A car stopped in front of the house. He heard his son's voice speaking to his mother. He could see the two of them; Tom had his arm around her. She was walking into the house now as if she had always meant to.

Mr. Cassidy lay back for the last moment of darkness. Soon the room would be full.

His son turned on the light.

People Like That
Are the Only People Here

Lorrie Moore

A beginning, an end: there seems to be neither. The whole thing is like a cloud that just lands, and everywhere inside it is full of rain. A start: the Mother finds a blood clot in the Baby's diaper. What is the story? Who put this here? It is big and bright, with a broken, khaki-colored vein in it. Over the weekend, the baby had looked listless and spacey, clayey and grim. But today he looks fine—so what is this thing, startling against the white diaper, like a tiny mouse heart packed in snow? Perhaps it belongs to someone else. Perhaps it is something menstrual, something belonging to the Mother or to the Babysitter, something the Baby has found in a wastebasket and for his own demented baby reasons stowed away here. (Babies—they're crazy! What can you do?) In her mind, the Mother takes this away from his body and attaches it to someone else's. There. Doesn't that make more sense?

Still, she phones the children's-hospital clinic. Blood in the diaper, she says, and, sounding alarmed and perplexed, the woman on the other end says, "Come in now."

Such pleasingly instant service! Just say "blood." Just say "diaper." Look what you get!

In the examination room, the pediatrician, the nurse, and the head resident all seem less alarmed and perplexed than simply per-plexed. At first, stupidly, the Mother is calmed by this. But soon, besides peering and saying "Hmm," the doctor, the nurse, and the head resident are all drawing their mouths in, bluish and tight—morning glories sensing noon. They fold their arms across their white-coated chests, unfold them again, and jot things down. They order an ultrasound. Bladder and kidneys. Here's the card. Go downstairs; turn left.

In Radiology, the Baby stands anxiously on the table, naked against the Mother, as she holds him still against her legs and waist, the Radiologist's cold scanning disk moving about the Baby's back. The Baby whimpers, looks up at the Mother. Let's get out of here, his eyes beg. Pick me up! The Radiologist stops, freezes one of the many swirls of oceanic gray, and clicks repeat-edly, a single moment within the long, cavernous weather map that is the Baby's insides.

"Are you finding something?" asks the Mother. Last year, her uncle Larry had a kidney removed for something that turned out to be benign. These imaging machines! They are like dogs, or metal detectors: they find everything but don't know what they've found. That's where the surgeons come in. They're like the owners of the dogs. Give me that, they say to the dog. What the heck is that?

"The surgeon will speak to you," says the Radiologist.

"Are you finding something?"

"The surgeon will speak to you," the Radiologist says again. "There seems to be something there, but the surgeon will talk to you about it."

"My uncle once had something on his kidney," says the Mother. "So they removed the kidney and it turned out the something was benign."

The Radiologist smiles a broad, ominous smile. "That's always the way it is," he says. "You don't know exactly what it is until it's in the bucket."

"In the bucket," the Mother repeats.

"That's doctor talk," the Radiologist says.

"It's very appealing," says the Mother. "It's a very appealing way to talk." Swirls of bile and blood, mustard and maroon in a pail, the colors of an African flag or some exuberant salad bar: in the bucket—she imagines it all.

The surgeon will see you soon," he says again. He tousles the Baby's ringlety hair. "Cute kid," he says.

"Let's see now," says the Surgeon, in one of his examining rooms. He has stepped in, then stepped out, then come back in again. He has crisp, frowning features, sharp bones, and a tennis-in-Bermuda tan. He crosses his blue-cottoned legs. He is wearing clogs.

The Mother knows her own face is a big white dumpling of worry. She is still wearing her long, dark parka, holding the Baby, who has pulled the hood up over her head because he always thinks it's funny to do that. Though on certain windy mornings she would like to think she could look vaguely romantic like this, like some French Lieutenant's Woman of the Prairie, in all her saner moments she knows she doesn't. She knows she looks ridiculous—like one of those animals made out of twisted party balloons. She lowers the hood and slips one arm out of the sleeve. The Baby wants to get up and play with the light switch. He fidgets, fusses, and points.

"He's big on lights these days," explains the Mother.

"That's O.K.," says the Surgeon, nodding toward the light switch. "Let him play with it." The Mother goes and stands by it, and the baby begins turning the lights off and on, off and on.

"What we have here is a Wilms' tumor," says the Surgeon, suddenly plunged into darkness. He says "tumor" as if it were the most normal thing in the world.

"Wilms'?" repeats the Mother. The room is quickly on fire again with light, then wiped dark again. Among the three of them here there is a long silence, as if it were suddenly the middle of the night. "Is that apostrophe 's' or 's' apostrophe?" the Mother says finally. She is a writer and a teacher. Spelling can be important— perhaps even at a time like this, though she has never before been at a time like this, so there are barbarisms she could easily commit without knowing.

The lights come on; the world is doused and exposed.

" 'S' apostrophe," says the Surgeon. "I think." The lights go back out, but the Surgeon continues speaking in the dark. "A malignant tumor of the left kidney."

Wait a minute. Hold on here. The Baby is only a baby, fed on organic applesauce and soy milk—a little prince!—and he was standing so close to her during the ultrasound. How could he have this terrible thing? It must have been her kidney. A fifties kidney. A DDT kidney. The Mother clears her throat. "Is it possible it was my kidney on the scan? I mean, I've never heard of a baby with a tumor, and, frankly, I was standing very close." She would make the blood hers, the tumor hers; it would all be some treacherous, farcical mistake.

"No, that's not possible," says the Surgeon. The light goes back on.

"It's not?" says the Mother. Wait until it's in the bucket, she thinks. Don't be so sure. Do we have to wait until it's in the bucket to find out a mistake has been made?

"We will start with a radical nephrectomy," says the Surgeon, instantly thrown into darkness again. His voice comes from nowhere and everywhere at once. "And then we'll begin with chemotherapy after that. These tumors usually respond very well to chemo."

"I've never heard of a baby having chemo," the Mother says. Baby and Chemo, she thinks: they should never even appear in the same sentence together, let alone the same life. In her other life, her life before this day, she was a believer in alternative medicine. Chemotherapy? Unthinkable. Now, suddenly, alternative medicine seems the wacko maiden aunt to the Nice Big Daddy of Conventional Treatment.

How quickly the old girl faints and gives way, leaves one just standing there. Chemo? Of course: chemo! Why, by all means: chemo. Absolutely! Chemo!

The Baby flicks the switch back on, and the walls reappear, big wedges of light checkered with small framed watercolors of the local lake. The Mother has begun to cry: all of life has led her here, to this moment. After this there is no more life. There is something else, something stumbling and unlivable, something mechanical, something for robots, but not life. Life has been taken and broken, quickly, like a stick. The room goes dark again, so that the Mother can cry more freely. How can a baby's body be stolen so fast? How much can one heaven-sent and unsuspecting child endure? Why has he not been spared this inconceivable fate?

Perhaps, she thinks, she is being punished: too many babysitters too early on. ("Come to Mommy! Come to Mommy-Babysitter!" she used to say. But it was a joke!) Her life, perhaps, bore too openly the marks and wigs of deepest drag. Her unmotherly thoughts had all been noted: the panicky hope that his nap would last just a little longer than it did; her occasional desire to kiss him passionately on the mouth (to make out with her baby!); her ongoing complaints about the very vocabulary of motherhood, how it degraded the speaker. ("Is this a poopie onesie? Yes, it's a very poopie onesie!") She had, moreover, on three occasions used the formula bottles as flower vases. She twice let the Baby's ears get fudgy with wax. A few afternoons last month, at snack time, she placed a bowl of Cheerios on the floor for him to eat, like a dog. She let him play with the Dust-buster. Just once, before he was born, she said, "Healthy? I just want the kid to be rich." A joke, for God's sake. After he was born, she announced that her life had become a daily sequence of mind-wrecking chores, the same ones over and over again, like a novel by Mrs. Camus. Another joke! These jokes will kill you. She had told too often, and with too much enjoyment, the story of how the Baby had said "Hi" to his high chair, waved at the lake waves, shouted "Goody-goody-goody" in what seemed to be a Russian accent, pointed at his eyes and said "Ice." And all that nonsensical baby talk: wasn't it a stitch? Canonical babbling, the language experts called it. He recounted whole stories in it, totally made up, she could tell; he embroidered, he fished, he exaggerated. What a card! To friends she spoke of his eating habits (carrots yes, tuna no). She mentioned, too much, his sidesplitting giggle. Did she have to be so boring? Did she have no consideration for others, for the intellectual demands and courtesies of human society? Would she not even attempt to be more interesting? It was a crime against the human mind not even to try.

Now her baby, for all these reasons—lack of motherly gratitude, motherly judgment, motherly proportion—will be taken away.

The room is fluorescently ablaze again. The Mother digs around in her parka pocket and comes up with a Kleenex. It is old and thin, like a mashed flower saved from a dance; she dabs it at her eyes and nose.

"The Baby won't suffer as much as you," says the Surgeon.

And who can contradict? Not the Baby, who in his Slavic Betty Boop voice can say only mama, dada, cheese, ice, bye-bye, out-side, boogie-boogie, goody-goody, eddy-eddy, and car. (Who is Eddy? They have no idea.) This will not suffice to express his mortal suffering. Who can say what babies do with their agony and shock? Not they themselves. (Baby talk: isn't it a stitch?) They put it all no place anyone can really see. They are like a different race, a different species: they seem not to experience pain the way we do. Yeah, that's it: their nervous systems are not as fully formed, and they just don't experience pain the way we do. A tune to keep one humming through the war. "You'll get through it," the Surgeon says.

"How?" asks the Mother. "How does one get through it?"

"You just put your head down and go," says the Surgeon. He picks up his file folder. He is a skilled manual laborer. The tricky emotional stuff is not to his liking. The babies. The babies! What can be said to console the parents about the babies? "I'll go phone the oncologist on duty to let him know," he says, and leaves the room.

"Come here, sweetie," the Mother says to the Baby, who has toddled off toward a gum wrapper on the floor. "We've got to put your jacket on." She picks him up and he reaches for the light switch again. Light, dark. Peekaboo: Where's baby? Where did baby go?

At home, she leaves a message—Urgent! Call me!—for the Husband on his voice mail. Then she takes the Baby upstairs for his nap, rocks him in the rocker. The Baby waves goodbye to his little bears, then looks toward the window and says, "Bye-bye, outside." He has, lately, the habit of waving goodbye to everything, and now it seems as if he sensed some imminent departure, and it breaks her heart to hear him. Bye-bye! She sings low and monotonously, like a small appliance, which is how he likes it. He is drowsy, dozy, drifting off. He has grown so much in the last year he hardly fits in her lap anymore; his limbs dangle off like a Pietà. His head rolls slightly inside the crook of her arm. She can feel him falling backward into sleep, his mouth round and open like the sweetest of poppies. All the lullabies in the world, all the melodies threaded through with maternal melancholy now become for her—abandoned as mothers can be by working men and napping babies—the songs of hard, hard grief. Sitting there, bowed and bobbing, the Mother feels the entirety of her love as worry and heartbreak. A quick and irrevocable alchemy: there is no longer one unworried scrap left for happiness. "If you go," she keens low into his soapy neck, into the ranunculus coil of his ear, "we are going with you. We are nothing without you. Without you, we are a heap of rocks. Without you, we are two stumps, with nothing any longer in our hearts. Wherever this takes you, we are following; we will be there. Don't be scared. We are going, too, wherever you go. That is that."

"Take notes," says the Husband, after coming straight home from work, midafternoon, hearing the news, and saying all the words out loud—surgery, metastasis, dialysis, transplant—then collapsing in a chair in tears. "Take notes. We are going to need money."

"Good God," cries the Mother. Everything inside her suddenly begins to cower and shrink, a thinning of bones. Perhaps this is a soldier's readiness, but it has the whiff of death and defeat. It feels like a heart attack, a failure of will and courage, a power failure: a failure of everything. Her face, when she glimpses it in a mirror, is cold and bloated with shock, her eyes scarlet and shrunk. She has already started to wear sunglasses indoors, like a celebrity widow. From where will her own strength come? From some philosophy? She is neither stalwart nor realistic and has trouble with basic concepts, such as the one that says events move in one direction only and do not jump up, turn around, and take themselves back.

The Husband begins too many of his sentences with "What if." He is trying to piece everything together, like a train wreck. He is trying to get the train to town.

"We'll just take all the steps, move through all the stages. We'll go where we have to go, we'll hunt, we'll find, we'll pay what we have to pay. What if we can't pay?"

"Sounds like shopping."

"I cannot believe this is happening to our little boy," he says, and starts to sob again.

What is to be said? You turn just slightly and there it is: the death of your child. It is part symbol, part devil, and in your blind spot all along, until it is upon you. Then it is a fierce little country abducting you; it holds you squarely inside itself like a cellar room—the best boundaries of you are the boundaries of it. Are there windows? Sometimes aren't there windows?

The Mother is not a shopper. She hates to shop, is generally bad at it, though she does like a good sale. She cannot stroll meaningfully through anger, denial, grief, and acceptance. She goes straight to bargaining and stays there. How much? She calls out to the ceiling, to some makeshift construction of holiness she has desperately though not uncreatively assembled in her mind and prayed to; a doubter, never before given to prayer, she must now reap what she has not sown; she must reassemble an entire altar of worship and begging. She tries for noble abstractions, nothing too anthropomorphic, just some Higher Morality, though if this particular Highness looks something like the manager at Marshall Field's, sucking a Frango mint, so be it. Amen. Just tell me what you want, requests the mother. And how do you want it? More charitable acts? A billion, starting now. Charitable thoughts? Harder, but of course! Of course! I'll do the cooking, honey, I'll pay the rent. Just tell me. Excuse me? Well, if not to you, to whom do I speak? Hello? To whom do I have to speak around here? A higher-up? A superior? Wait? I can wait. I've got the whole damn day.

The Husband now lies next to her on their bed, sighing. "Poor little guy could survive all this only to be killed in a car crash at the age of sixteen," he says.

The Mother, bargaining, considers this. "We'll take the car crash," she says.

"What?"

"Let's Make a Deal! Sixteen is a full life! We'll take the car crash. We'll take the car crash in front of which Carol Merrill is now standing."

Now the Manager of Marshall Field's reappears. "To take the surprises out is to take the life out of life," he says.

The phone rings. The Husband leaves the room.

"But I don't want these surprises," says the Mother. "Here! You take these surprises!"

"To know the narrative in advance is to turn yourself into a machine," the Manager continues. "What makes humans human is precisely that they do not know the future. That is why they do the fateful and amusing things they do: who can say how anything will turn out? Therein lies the only hope for redemption, discovery, and—let's be frank—fun, fun, fun! There might be things people will get away with. And not just motel towels. There might be great illicit loves, enduring joy—or faith-shaking accidents with farm machinery. But you have to not know in order to see what stories your life's efforts bring you. The mystery is all."

The Mother, though shy, has grown confrontational. "Is this the kind of bogus, random crap they teach at merchandising school? We would like fewer surprises, fewer efforts and mysteries, thank you. K through 8; can we just get K through 8?" It now seems like the luckiest, most beautiful, most musical phrase she's ever heard: K through 8—the very lilt. The very thought.

The Manager continues, trying things out. "I mean, the whole concept of 'the story,' of cause and effect, the whole idea that people have a clue as to how the world works, is just a piece of laughable metaphysical colonialism perpetrated upon the wild country of time."

Did they own a gun? The Mother begins looking through drawers.

The Husband comes back in the room and observes her. "Ha! The Great Havoc That Is the Puzzle of All Life!" he says of the Marshall Field's management policy. He has just gotten off a conference call with the insurance company and the hospital. The surgery will be Friday. "It's all just some dirty capitalist's idea of a philosophy."

"Maybe it's just a fact of narrative, and you really can't politicize it," says the Mother. It is now only the two of them.

"Whose side are you on?"

"I'm on the Baby's side."

"Are you taking notes for this?"

"No."

"You're not?"

"No. I can't. Not this! I write fiction. This isn't fiction."

"Then write nonfiction. Do a piece of journalism. Get two dollars a word."

"Then it has to be true and full of information. I'm not trained. I'm not that skilled. Plus, I have a convenient personal principle about artists' not abandoning art. One should never turn one's back on a vivid imagination. Even the whole memoir thing annoys me."

"Well, make things up but pretend they're real."

"I'm not that insured."

"You're making me nervous."

"Sweetie, darling, I'm not that good. I can't do this. I can do—what can I do? I can do quasi-amusing phone dialogue. I can do succinct descriptions of weather. I can do screwball outings with the family pet. Sometimes I can do those. Honey, I only do what I can. I do the careful ironies of daydream. I do the marshy ideas upon which intimate life is built. But this? Our baby with cancer? I'm sorry. My stop was two stations back. This is irony at its most gaudy and careless. This is a Hieronymus Bosch of facts and figures and blood and graphs. This is a night-mare of narrative slop. This cannot be designed. This cannot even be noted in preparation for a design—"

"We're going to need the money."

"To say nothing of the moral boundaries of pecuniary recompense in a situation such as this—"

"What if the other kidney goes? What if he needs a transplant? Where are the moral boundaries there? What are we going to do, have bake sales?"

"We can sell the house. I hate this house. It makes me crazy."

"And we'll live—where again?"

"The Ronald McDonald place. I hear it's nice. It's the least McDonald's can do."

"You have a keen sense of justice."

"I try. What can I say?"

The Husband buries his face in his hands: "Our poor baby. How did this happen to him?" He looks over and stares at the bookcase that serves as their nightstand. "And is any one of these baby books a help?" He picks up the Leach, the Spock, the "What to Expect." "Where in the pages or index of any of these does it say 'chemotherapy' or 'Hickman catheter' or 'renal sarcoma'? Where does it say 'carcinogenesis' or 'metastasis'? You know what these books are obsessed with? Holding a fucking spoon." He begins hurling the books off the nightstand and against the far wall.

"Hey," says the Mother, trying to soothe. "Hey, hey, hey." But, compared with his stormy roar, her words are those of a backup singer—a Shondell, a Pip—a doo-wop ditty. Books, and now more books, continue to fly.

TAKE NOTES. Is "fainthearted" one word or two? Student prose has wrecked her spelling.

It's one word. Two words—faint hearted—what would that be? The name of a drag queen.

TAKE NOTES. In the end you suffer alone. But at the beginning you suffer with a whole lot of others. When your child has cancer you are instantly whisked away to another planet: one of bald-headed little boys. Pediatric Oncology. Peed-Onk. You wash your hands for thirty seconds in antibacterial soap before you are allowed to enter through the swinging doors. You put paper slippers on your shoes. You keep your voice down. "Almost all the children are boys," one of the nurses says. "No one knows why. It's been documented, but a lot of people out there still don't realize it." The little boys are all from sweet-sounding places, Janesville and Appleton—little heartland towns with giant landfills, agricultural runoff, paper factories, Joe McCarthy's grave. (Alone a site of great toxicity, thinks the Mother. The soil should be tested.)

All the bald little boys look like brothers. They wheel their I.V.s up and down the single corridor of Peed-Onk. Some of the lively ones, feeling good for a day, ride the lower bars of their I.V.s while their large, cheerful mothers whizz them along the halls. Wheee!

The Mother does not feel large and cheerful. In her mind she is scathing, acid-tongued, wraith-thin, and chain-smoking out on a fire escape somewhere. Below her lie the gentle undulations of the Midwest, with all its aspirations to be—to be what? To be Long Island. How it has succeeded! Strip mall upon strip mall. Lurid water, poisoned potatoes. The Mother drags deeply, blowing clouds of smoke out over the disfigured cornfields. When a baby gets cancer, it seems stupid ever to have given up smoking. When a baby gets cancer, you think, Whom are we kidding? Let's all light up. When a baby gets cancer, you think, Who came up with this idea? Pour me a drink so I can refuse to toast.

The Mother does not know how to be one of these other mothers, with their blond hair and sweatpants and sneakers and determined pleasantness. She does not think that she can be anything similar. She does not feel remotely like them. She knows, for instance, too many people in Greenwich Village. She mail-orders oysters and tiramisù from a shop in SoHo. She is close friends with four actual homosexuals. Her husband is asking her to Take Notes.

Where do these women get their sweatpants? She will find out.

She will start, perhaps, with the costume and work from there.

She will live according to the bromides: Take one day at a time. Take a positive attitude. Take a hike! She wishes that there were more interesting things that were useful and true, but it seems now that it's only the boring things that are useful and true. One day at a time. And At least we have our health. How ordinary. How obvious. One day at a time: you need a brain for that?

While the Surgeon is fine-boned, regal, and laconic—they have correctly guessed his game to be doubles—there is a bit of the mad, over-caffeinated scientist to the Oncologist. He speaks quickly. He knows a lot of studies and numbers. He can do the math. Good! Someone should be able to do the math! "It's a fast but wimpy tumor," he explains. "It typically metastasizes to the lung." He rattles off some numbers, time frames, risk statistics. Fast but wimpy: the Mother tries to imagine this combination of traits, tries to think and think, and can only come up with Claudia Osk from the fourth grade, who blushed and almost wept when called on in class but in gym could outrun everyone in the quarter-mile, fire-door-to-fence dash. The Mother thinks now of this tumor as Claudia Osk. They are going to get Claudia Osk, make her sorry. All right! Claudia Osk must die. Though it has never been mentioned before, it now seems clear that Claudia Osk should have died long ago. Who was she, anyway? So conceited, not letting anyone beat her in a race. Well, hey, hey, hey—don't look now, Claudia!

The Husband nudges her. "Are you listening?"

"The chances of this happening even just to one kidney are one in fifteen thousand. Now, given all these other factors, the chances on the second kidney are about one in eight."

"One in eight," says the Husband. "Not bad. As long as it's not one in fifteen thousand."

The Mother studies the trees and fish along the ceiling's edge in the Save the Planet wallpaper border. Save the Planet. Yes! But the windows in this very building don't open, and diesel fumes are leaking into the ventilating system, near which, outside, a delivery truck is parked. The air is nauseous and stale.

"Really," the Oncologist is saying, "of all the cancers he could get, this is probably one of the best."

"We win," says the Mother.

" 'Best', I know, hardly seems the right word. Look, you two probably need to get some rest. We'll see how the surgery and histology go. Then we'll start with chemo the week following. A little light chemo: vincristine and—"

"Vincristine?" interrupts the Mother. "Wine of Christ?"

"The names are strange, I know. The other one we use is actinomycin-D. Sometimes called dactinomycin. People move the 'D' around to the front."

"They move the 'D' around to the front," repeats the Mother.

"Yup," the Oncologist says. "I don't know why, they just do!"

"Christ didn't survive his wine," says the Husband.

"But of course he did," says the Oncologist and nods toward the Baby, who has now found a cupboard full of hospital linens and bandages and is yanking them all out onto the floor. "I'll see you guys tomorrow, after the surgery." And with that the Oncologist leaves.

"Or, rather, Christ was his wine," mumbles the Husband. Everything he knows about the New Testament he has gleaned from the soundtrack of "Godspell." "His blood was the wine. What a great beverage idea."

"A little light chemo. Don't you like that one?" says the Mother. "Eine kleine dactinomycin. I'd like to see Mozart write that one up for a big wad o' cash."

"Come here, honey," the Husband says to the Baby, who has now pulled off both his shoes.

"It's bad enough when they refer to medical science as an inexact science," says the Mother. "But when they start referring to it as an art I get extremely nervous."

"Yeah. If we wanted art, Doc, we'd go to an art museum." The Husband picks up the Baby. "You're an artist," he says to the Mother with the taint of accusation in his voice. "They probably think you find creativity reassuring."

The Mother sighs. "I just find it inevitable. Let's go get something to eat." And so they take the elevator to the cafeteria, where there is a high chair, and where, not noticing, they all eat a lot of apples with the price tags still on them.

Because his surgery is not until tomorrow, the Baby likes the hospital. He likes the long corridors, down which he can run. He likes everything on wheels. The flower carts in the lobby! ("Please keep your boy away from the flowers," says the vender. "We'll buy the whole display," snaps the Mother, adding, "Actual children in a children's hospital—unbelievable, isn't it?") The Baby likes the other little boys. Places to go! People to see! Rooms to wander into! There is Intensive Care. There is the Trauma Unit. The Baby smiles and waves. What a little Cancer Personality! Bandaged citizens smile and wave back. In Peed-Onk there are the bald little boys to play with. Joey, Eric, Tim, Mort, and Tod. (Mort! Tod!) There is the four-year-old, Ned, holding his little deflated rubber ball, the one with the intriguing curling hose. The Baby wants to play with it. "It's mine, leave it alone," says Ned. "Tell the baby to leave it alone."

"Baby, you've got to share," says the mother from a chair some feet away.

Suddenly, from down near the Tiny Tim Lounge, comes Ned's mother, large and blonde and sweatpanted. "Stop that! Stop It!" she cries out, dashing toward the Baby and Ned and pushing the Baby away. "Don't touch that!" she barks at the Baby, who is only a baby and bursts into tears because he has never been yelled at like this before.

Ned's mom glares at everyone. "This is drawing fluid from Neddy's liver!" She pats at the rubber thing and starts to cry a little.

"Oh my God," says the Mother. She comforts the Baby, who is also crying. She and Ned, the only dry-eyed people, look at each other. "I'm so sorry," she says to Ned and then to his mother. "I'm so stupid. I thought they were squabbling over a toy."

"It does look like a toy," agrees Ned. He smiles. He is an angel. All the little boys are angels. Total, sweet, bald little angels, and now God is trying to get them back for himself. Who are they, mere mortal women, in the face of this, this powerful and overwhelming and inscrutable thing, God's will? They are the mothers, that's who. You can't have him! they shout every day. You dirty old man! Get out of here! Hands off!

"I'm so sorry," says the Mother again. "I didn't know."

Ned's mother smiles vaguely. "Of course you didn't know," she says, and walks back to the Tiny Tim Lounge.

The Tiny Tim Lounge is a little sitting area at the end of the Peed-Onk corridor. There are two small sofas, a table, a rocking chair, a television, and a VCR. There are various videos: "Speed," "Dune," "Star Wars." On one of the lounge walls there is a gold plaque with the musician Tiny Tim's name on it: years ago, his son was treated at this hospital, and so he donated money for this lounge. It is a cramped little lounge, which one suspects would be larger if Tiny Tim's son had actually lived. Instead, he died here, at this hospital, and now there is this tiny room which is part gratitude, part generosity, part Fuck-you.

Sifting through the videocassettes, the Mother wonders what science fiction could begin to compete with the science fiction of cancer itself: a tumor, with its differentiated muscle and bone cells, a clump of wild nothing and its mad, ambitious desire to be something—something inside you, instead of you, another organism but with a monster's architecture, a demon's sabotage and chaos: Think of leukemia, a tumor diabolically taking liquid form, the better to swim about incognito in the blood. George Lucas, direct that!

Sitting with the other parents in the Tiny Tim Lounge, the night before the surgery, having put the Baby to bed in his high steel crib two rooms down, the Mother begins to hear the stories: leukemia in kindergarten, sarcomas in Little League, neuroblastomas discovered at summer camp. Eric slid into third base, but then the scrape didn't heal. The parents pat one another's forearms and speak of other children's hospitals as if they were resorts. "You were at St. Jude's last winter? So were we. What did you think of it? We loved the staff." Jobs have been quit, marriages hacked up, bank accounts ravaged; the parents have seemingly endured the unendurable. They speak not of the possibility of comas brought on by the chemo but of the number of them. "He was in his first coma last July," says Ned's mother. "It was a scary time, but we pulled through."

Pulling through is what people do around here. There is a kind of bravery in their lives that isn't bravery at all. It is automatic, unflinching, a mix of man and machine, consuming and unquestionable obligation meeting illness move for move in a giant, even-Steven game of chess: an unending round of something that looks like shadowboxing—though between love and death, which is the shadow? "Everyone admires us for our courage," says one man. "They have no idea what they're talking about."

I could get out of here, thinks the Mother. I could just get on a bus and go, never come back. Change my name. A kind of witness relocation thing.

"Courage requires options," the man adds.

The Baby might be better off.

"There are options," says a woman with a thick suède head-band. "You could give up. You could fall apart."

"No, you can't. Nobody does. I've never seen it," says the man. "Well, not really fall apart." Then the lounge is quiet. Over the VCR someone has taped the fortune from a fortune cookie. Optimism, it says, is what allows a teakettle to sing though up to its neck in hot water. Underneath, someone else has taped a clipping from a summer horoscope. Cancer rules! it says. Who would tape this up? Somebody's twelve-year-old brother. One of the fathers—Joey's father—gets up and tears them both off, makes a small wad in his fist.

There is some rustling of magazine pages.

The Mother clears her throat. "Tiny Tim forgot the wet bar," she says.

Ned, who is still up, comes out of his room and down the corridor, whose lights dim at nine. Standing next to the Mother's chair, he says to her, "Where are you from? What is wrong with your baby?"

In the little room that is theirs, she sleeps fitfully in her sweatpants, occasionally leaping up to check on the Baby. This is what the sweatpants are for: leaping. In case of fire. In case of anything. In case the difference between day and night starts to dissolve and there is no difference at all so why pretend. In the cot beside her the Husband, who has taken a sleeping pill, is snoring loudly, his arms folded about his head in a kind of origami. How could either of them have stayed at the house, with its empty high chair and empty crib? Occasionally the Baby wakes and cries out, and she bolts up, goes to him, rubs his back, rearranges linens. The clock on the metal dresser shows that it is five after three. Then twenty to five. And then it is really morning, the beginning of this day, Nephrectomy Day. Will she be glad when it's over, or barely alive, or both? Each day of this week has arrived huge, empty, and unknown, like a spaceship, and this one especially is lit an incandescent gray.

"He'll need to put this on," says John, one of the nurses, bright and early, handing the Mother a thin greenish garment with roses and Teddy bears printed on it. A wave of nausea hits her: this smock, she thinks, will soon be splattered with—with what?

The Baby is awake but drowsy. She lifts off his pajamas. "Don't forget, bubeleh," she whispers, undressing and dressing him. "We will be with you every moment, every step. When you think you are asleep and floating off far away from everybody, Mommy will still be there." If she hasn't fled on a bus. "Mommy will take care of you. And Daddy, too." She hopes the Baby does not detect her own fear and uncertainty, which she must hide from him, like a limp. He is hungry, not having been allowed to eat, and he is no longer amused by this new place but worried about its hardships. Oh, my baby, she thinks. And the room starts to swim a little. The Husband comes in to take over. "Take a break," he says to her. "I'll walk him around for five minutes."

She leaves but doesn't know where to go. In the hallway she is approached by a kind of social worker, a customer-relations person, who had given them a video to watch about the anesthesia: how the parent accompanies the child into the operating room, and how gently, nicely the drugs are administered.

"Did you watch the video?"

"Yes," says the Mother.

"Wasn't it helpful?"

"I don't know," says the Mother.

"Do you have any questions?" asks the video woman. Do you have any questions? asked of someone who has recently landed in this fearful, alien place seems to the Mother an absurd and amazing little courtesy. The very specificity of a question would give the lie to the overwhelming strangeness of everything around her.

"Not right now," says the Mother. "Right now I think I'm just going to go to the bathroom."

When she comes back to the Baby's room, everyone is there: the Surgeon, the Anesthesiologist, all the nurses, the social worker. In their blue caps and scrubs, they look like a clutch of forget-me-nots, and forget them who could? The Baby, in his little Teddy-bear smock, seems cold and scared. He reaches out and the Mother lifts him from the Husband's arms, rubs his back to warm him.

"Well, it's time!" says the Surgeon, forcing a smile.

"Shall we go?" says the Anesthesiologist.

What follows is a blur of obedience and bright lights. They take an elevator down to a big concrete room, the anteroom, the greenroom, the backstage of the operating room. Lining the walls are long shelves full of blue surgical outfits. "Children often become afraid of the color blue," one of the nurses says. But of course. Of course! "Now, which one of you would like to come into the operating room for the anesthesia?"

"I will," says the Mother.

"Are you sure?" asks the Husband.

"Yup." She kisses the Baby's hair. Mr. Curlyhead people keep calling him here, and it seems both rude and nice. Women look admiringly at his long lashes and exclaim, "Always the boys! Always the boys!"

Two surgical nurses put a blue smock and a blue cotton cap on the Mother. The Baby finds this funny and keeps pulling at the cap. "This way," says another nurse, and the Mother follows. "Just put the Baby down on the table."

In the video, the mother holds the baby and fumes from the mask are gently waved under the baby's nose until he falls asleep. Now, out of view of camera or social worker, the Anesthesiologist is anxious to get this under way and not let too much gas leak out into the room generally. The occupational hazard of this, his chosen profession, is gas exposure and nerve damage, and it has started to worry him. No doubt he frets about it to his wife every night. Now he turns the gas on and quickly clamps the plastic mouthpiece over the baby's cheeks and lips.

The Baby is startled. The Mother is startled. The Baby starts to scream and redden behind the plastic, but he cannot be heard. He thrashes. "Tell him it's O.K.," says the nurse to the Mother.

O.K.? "It's O.K.," repeats the Mother, holding his hand, but she knows he can tell it's not O.K., because he can see that not only is she still wearing that stupid paper cap but her words are mechanical and swallowed, and she is biting her lips to keep them from trembling. Panicked, he attempts to sit, he cannot breathe, his arms reach up. Bye-bye, outside. And then, quite quickly, his eyes shut; he untenses and has fallen not into sleep but aside to sleep, an odd, kidnapping kind of sleep, his terror now hidden someplace deep inside him.

"How did it go?" asks the social worker, waiting in the concrete outer room. The Mother is hysterical. A nurse has ushered her out.

"It wasn't at all like the film strip!" she cries. "It wasn't like the film strip at all!"

"The film strip? You mean the video?" asks the social worker.

"It wasn't like that at all! It was brutal and unforgivable."

"Why that's terrible," she says, her role now no longer misinformational but janitorial, and she touches the Mother's arm. The Mother shakes her off and goes to find the Husband.

She finds him in the large mulberry Surgery Lounge, where he has been taken and where there is free hot chocolate in small plastic-foam cups. Red cellophane garlands festoon the doorways. She has totally forgotten it is as close to Christmas as this. A pianist in the corner is playing "Carol of the Bells," and it sounds not only unfestive but scary, like the theme from *The Exorcist*.

There is a giant clock on the far wall. It is a kind of porthole into the operating room, a way of assessing the Baby's ordeal: forty-five minutes for the Hickman implant; two and a half hours for the nephrectomy. And then, after that, three months of chemotherapy. The magazine on her lap stays open at a ruby-hued perfume ad.

"Still not taking notes," says the Husband.

"Nope."

"You know, in a way, this is the kind of thing you've always written about."

"You are really something, you know that? This is life. This isn't a 'kind of thing.'"

"But this is the kind of thing that fiction is: it's the unlivable life, the strange room tacked on to the house, the extra moon that is circling the earth unbeknownst to science."

"I told you that."

"I'm quoting you."

She looks at her watch, thinking of the Baby. "How long has it been?"

"Not long. Too long. In the end, those're the same things."

"What do you suppose is happening to him right this second?"

Infection? Slipping knives? "I don't know. But you know what? I've gotta go. I've gotta just walk a bit." The Husband gets up, walks around the lounge, then comes back and sits down.

The synapses between the minutes are unswimmable. An hour is thick as fudge. The Mother feels depleted; she is a string of empty tin cans attached by wire, something a goat would sniff and chew, something now and then enlivened by a jolt of electricity.

She hears their names being called over the intercom. "Yes? Yes?" She stands up quickly. Her voice has flown out before her, an exhalation of birds. The piano music has stopped. The pianist is gone. She and the Husband approach the main desk, where a man looks up at them and smiles. Before him is a Xeroxed list of patients' names. "That's our little boy right there," says the Mother, seeing the Baby's name on the list and pointing at it. "Is there some word? Is everything O.K.?"

"Yes," says the man. "Your boy is doing fine. They've just finished with the catheter and they are moving on to the kidney."

"But it's been two hours already! Oh, my God, did something go wrong, what happened, what went wrong?"

"Did something go wrong?" The Husband tugs at his collar.

"Not really. It just took longer than they expected. I'm told everything is fine. They wanted you to know."

"Thank you," says the Husband. They turn and walk back toward where they were sitting.

"I'm not going to make it," sighs the Mother, sinking into a fake-leather chair shaped somewhat like a baseball mitt. "But before I go I'm taking half this hospital out with me."

"Do you want some coffee?" asks the Husband.

"I don't know," says the Mother. "No, I guess not. No. Do you?"

"Nah, I don't, either, I guess," he says.

"Would you like part of an orange?"

"Oh, maybe, I guess, if you're having one." She takes a temple orange from her purse and just sits there peeling its difficult skin, the flesh rupturing beneath her fingers, the juice trickling down her hands, stinging the hangnails. She and the Husband chew and swallow, discreetly spit the seeds into Kleenex, and read from photocopies of the latest medical research which they begged from the interne. They read, and underline, and sigh and close their eyes, and after some time the surgery is over. A nurse from Peed-Onk comes down to tell them.

"Your little boy's in recovery right now. He's doing well. You can see him in about fifteen minutes."

How can it be described? How can any of it be described? The trip and the story of the trip are always two different things. The narrator is the one who has stayed home but then, afterward, presses her mouth upon the traveller's mouth, in order to make the mouth work, to make the mouth say, say, say. One cannot go to a place and speak of it, one cannot both see and say, not really. One can go, and upon returning make a lot of hand motions and indications with the arms. The mouth itself, working at the speed of light, at the eye's instructions, is necessarily struck still; so fast, so much to report, it hangs open and dumb as a gutted bell.

All that unsayable life! That's where the narrator comes in. The narrator comes with her kisses and mimicry and tidying up. The narrator comes and makes a slow, fake song of the mouth's eager devastation.

It is a horror and a miracle to see him. He is lying in his crib in his room, tubed up, splayed like a boy on a cross, his arms stiffened into cardboard "no-no's" so that he cannot yank out the tubes. There is the bladder catheter, the nasal-gastric tube, and the Hickman, which, beneath the skin, is plugged into his jugular, then popped out his chest wall and capped with a long plastic cap. There is a large bandage taped over his abdomen. Groggy, on a morphine drip, still he is able to look at her when, maneuvering through all the vinyl wiring, she leans to hold him, and when she does he begins to cry, but cry silently, without motion or noise. She has never seen a baby cry without motion or noise. It is the crying of an old person: silent, beyond opinion, shattered. In someone so tiny, it is frightening and unnatural. She wants to pick up the Baby and run—out of there, out of there. She wants to whip out a gun: No-no's, eh? This whole thing is what I call a no-no. "Don't you touch him!" she wants to shout at the surgeons and the needle nurses. "Not anymore! No more! No more!" She would crawl up and lie beside him in the crib if she could. But instead, because of all his intricate wiring, she must lean and cuddle, sing to him, songs of peril and flight: "We gotta get out of this place, if it's the last thing we ever do. We gotta get out of this place. Baby, there's a better life for me and you."

Very 1967. She was eleven then, and impressionable.

The Baby looks at her, pleadingly, his arms outstretched in surrender. To where? Where is there to go? Take me! Take me!

That night, post-op night, the Mother and the Husband lie afloat in their cots. A fluorescent lamp near the crib is kept on in the dark. The Baby breathes evenly but thinly in his drugged sleep. The morphine in its first flooding doses apparently makes him feel as if he were falling backward—or so the Mother has been told— and it causes the Baby to jerk, to catch himself over and over, as if he were being dropped from a tree. "Is this right? Isn't there something that should be done?" The nurses come in hourly, different ones—the night shifts seem strangely short and frequent. If the Baby stirs or frets, the nurses give him more morphine through the Hickman catheter, then leave to tend to other patients. The Mother rises to check on him herself in the low light. There is gurgling from the clear plastic suction tube coming out of his mouth. Brownish clumps have collected in the tube. What is going on? The Mother rings for the nurse. Is it Renee or Sarah or Darcy? She's forgotten.

"What, what is it?" murmurs the Husband, waking up.

"Something is wrong," says the Mother. "It looks like blood in his N-G tube."

"What?" The Husband gets out of bed. He, too, is wearing sweatpants.

The nurse—Valerie—pushes open the heavy door to the room and enters quietly. "Everything O.K.?"

"There's something wrong here. The tube is sucking blood out of his stomach. It looks like it may have perforated his stomach and now he's bleeding internally. Look!"

Valerie is a saint, but her voice is the standard hospital saint voice: an infuriating, pharmaceutical calm. It says, Everything is normal here. Death is normal. Pain is normal. Nothing is abnormal. So there is nothing to get excited about. "Well, now, let's see." She holds up the plastic tube and tries to see inside it. "Hmm," she says. "I'll call the attending physician."

Because this is a research and teaching hospital, all the regular doctors are at home sleeping in their Mission-style beds. Tonight, as is apparently the case every weekend night, the attending physician is a medical student. He looks fifteen. The authority he attempts to convey he cannot remotely inhabit. He is not even in the same building with it. He shakes everyone's hand, then strokes his chin, a gesture no doubt gleaned from some piece of dinner theatre his parents took him to once. As if there were an actual beard on that chin! As if beard growth on that chin were even possible! "Our Town"! "Kiss Me Kate"! "Barefoot in the Park"! He is attempting to convince if not to impress.

"We're in trouble," the Mother whispers to the Husband. She is tired, tired of young people grubbing for grades. "We've got Dr. 'Kiss Me Kate' here."

The Husband looks at her blankly, a mixture of disorientation and divorce.

The medical student holds the tubing in both hands. "I don't really see anything," he says.

He flunks! "You don't?" The Mother shoves her way in, holds the clear tubing in both hands. "That," she says. "Right her and here." Just this past semester she said to one of her own students, "If you don't see how this essay is better than that one, then I want you to just go out into the hallway and stand there until you do." Is it important to keep one's voice down? The Baby stays asleep. He is drugged and dreaming, far away.

"Hmm," says the medical student. "Perhaps there's a little irritation in the stomach."

"A little irritation?" The Mother grows furious. "This is blood. These are clumps and clots. This stupid thing is sucking the life right out of him!" Life! She is starting to cry.

They turn off the suction and bring in antacids, which they feed into the Baby through the tube. Then they turn the suction on again. This time on "low."

"What was it on before?" asks the Husband.

"High," says Valerie. "Doctor's orders, though I don't know why. I don't know why these doctors do a lot of the things they do."

"Maybe they're—not all that bright?" suggests the Mother. She is feeling relief and rage simultaneously: there is a feeling of prayer and litigation in the air. Yet essentially she is grateful. Isn't she? She thinks she is. And still, and still: look at all the things you have to do to protect a child, a hospital merely an intensification of life's cruel obstacle course.

The Surgeon comes to visit on Saturday morning. He steps in and nods at the Baby, who is awake but glazed from the morphine, his eyes two dark, unseeing grapes. "The boy looks fine," he announces. He peeks under the Baby's bandage. "The stitches look good," he says. The Baby's abdomen is stitched all the way across, like a baseball. "And the other kidney, when we looked at it yesterday face to face, looked fine. We'll try to wean him off the morphine a little, and see how he's doing on Monday."

"Is he going to be O.K.?"

"The boy? The boy is going to be fine," he says, then taps her stiffly on the shoulder. "Now, you take care. It's Saturday. Drink a little wine."

Over the weekend, while the Baby sleeps, the Mother and the Husband sit together in the Tiny Tim Lounge. The Husband is restless and makes cafeteria and sundry runs, running errands for everyone. In his absence, the other parents regale her further with their sagas. Pediatric cancer and chemo stories: the children's amputations, blood poisoning, teeth flaking like shale, the learning delays and disabilities caused by chemo frying the young, budding brain. But strangely optimistic codas are tacked on: endings as stiff and loopy as carpenter's lace, crisp and empty as lettuce, reticulate as a net—ah, words. "After all that business with the tumor, he's better now, and fitted with new incisors by my wife's cousin's husband, who did dental school in two and a half years, if you can believe that. We hope for the best. We take things as they come. Life is hard."

"Life's a big problem," agrees the Mother. Part of her welcomes and invites all their tales. In the few long days since this nightmare began, part of her has become addicted to disaster and war stories. She only wants to hear about the sadness and emergencies of others. They are the only situations that can join hands with her own; everything else bounces off her shiny shield of resentment and unsympathy. Nothing else can even stay in her brain. From this, no doubt, the philistine world is made, or should one say recruited? Together the parents huddle all day in the Tiny Tim Lounge—no need to watch "Oprah." They leave "Oprah" in the dust. "Oprah" has nothing on them. They chat matter-of-factly, then fall silent and watch "Dune" or "Star Wars," in which there are bright and shiny robots, whom the Mother now sees not as robots at all but as human beings who have had terrible things happen to them.

Some of their friends visit with stuffed animals and soft "Looking good"'s for the dozing baby, though the room is way past the stuffed-animal limit. The Mother arranges, once more, a plateful of Mint Milano cookies and cups of takeout coffee for guests. All her nutso pals stop by—the two on Prozac, the one obsessed with the word "penis" in the word "happiness," the one who recently had her hair foiled green. "Your friends put the de in fin de siècle," says the Husband. Overheard, or recorded, all marital conversation sounds as if someone must be joking, though usually no one is.

She loves her friends, especially loves them for coming, since there are times they all fight and don't speak for weeks. Is this friendship? For now and here, it must do and is, and is, she swears it is. For one, they never offer impromptu spiritual lectures about death, how it is part of life, its natural ebb and flow, how we all must accept that, or other such utterances that make her want to scratch out somebody's eyes. Like true friends, they take no hardy or elegant stance loosely choreographed from some broad perspective. They get right in there and mutter "Jesus Christ!" and shake their heads. Plus, they are the only people who not only will laugh at her stupid jokes but offer up stupid ones of their own. What do you get when you cross Tiny Tim with a pit bull? A child's illness is a strain on the mind. They know how to laugh in a flutey, desperate way—unlike the people who are more her husband's friends and who seem just to deepen their sorrowful gazes, nodding their heads in Sympathy. How Exiling and Estranging are everybody's Sympathetic Expressions! When anyone laughs, she thinks, O.K. Hooray! A buddy. In disaster as in show business.

Nurses come and go; their chirpy voices both startle and soothe. Some of the other Peed-Onk parents stick their heads in to see how the Baby is and offer encouragement.

Green Hair scratches her head. "Everyone's so friendly here. Is there someone in this place who isn't doing all this airy, scripted optimism—or are people like that the only people here?"

"It's Modern Middle Medicine meets the Modern Middle Family," says the Husband. "In the Modern Middle West."

Someone has brought in takeout lo mein, and they all eat it out in the hall by the elevators.

Parents are allowed use of the Courtesy Line.

"You've got to have a second child," says a friend on the phone, a friend from out of town. "An heir and a spare. That's what we did. We had another child to insure we wouldn't off ourselves if we lost our first."

"Really?"

"I'm serious."

"A formal suicide? Wouldn't you just drink yourself into a lifelong stupor and let it go at that?"

"Nope. I knew how I would do it even. For a while, until our second came along, I had it all planned."

"You did? What did you plan?"

"I can't go into too much detail, because—hi honey!—the kids are here now in the room. But I'll spell out the general idea: R-O-P-E."

Sunday evening she goes and sinks down on the sofa in the Tiny Tim Lounge next to Frank, Joey's father. He is a short, stocky man with the currentless, flat-lined look behind the eyes that all the parents eventually get here. He has shaved his head bald in solidarity with his son. His little boy has been battling cancer for five years. It is now in the liver, and the rumor around the corridor is that Joey has three weeks to live. She knows that Joey's mother, Roseanne, left Frank years ago, two years into the cancer, and has remarried and had another child, a girl named Brittany. The Mother sees Roseanne here sometimes with her new life—the cute little girl and the new full-haired husband, who will never be so maniacally and debilitatingly obsessed with Joey's illness the way Frank, her first husband, is.

Roseanne comes to visit Joey, to say hello and now goodbye, but she is not Joey's main man. Frank is.

Frank is full of stories—about the doctors, about the food, about the nurses, about Joey. Joey, affectless from his meds, sometimes leaves his room and comes out to watch TV in his bathrobe. He is jaundiced and bald, and though he is nine he looks no older than six. Frank has devoted the last four and a half years to saving Joey's life. When the cancer was first diagnosed, the doctors gave Joey a twenty-per-cent chance of living six more months. Now here it is almost five years later, and Joey's still here. It is all due to Frank, who, early on, quit his job as vice-president of a consulting firm in order to commit himself totally to his son. He is proud of everything he's given up and done, but he is tired. Part of him now really believes that things are coming to a close, that this is the end. He says this without tears. There are no more tears.

"You have probably been through more than anyone else on this corridor," says the Mother.

"I could tell you stories," he says. There is a sour odor between them, and she realizes that neither of them has bathed for days.

"Tell me one. Tell me the worst one." She knows he hates his ex-wife and hates her new husband even more.

"The worst? They're all the worst. Here's one: one morning I went out for breakfast with my buddy—it was the only time I'd left Joey alone ever, left him for two hours is all—and when I came back his N-G tube was full of blood. They had the suction on too high, and it was sucking the guts right out of him."

"Oh, my God. That just happened to us," said the Mother.

"It did?"

"Friday night."

"You're kidding. They let that happen again? I gave them such a chewing out about that!"

"I guess our luck is not so good. We get your very worst story on the second night we're here."

"It's not a bad place, though."

"It's not?"

"Naw. I've seen worse. I've taken Joey everywhere."

"He seems very strong." Truth is, at this point Joey seems like a zombie and frightens her.

"Joey's a fucking genius. A biological genius. They'd given him six months, remember."

The Mother nods.

"Six months is not very long," says Frank. "Six months is nothing. He was four and a half years old."

All the words are like blows. She feels flooded with affection and mourning for this man. She looks away, out the window, out past the hospital parking lot, up toward the black marbled sky and the electric eyelash of the moon. "And now he's nine," she says. "You're his hero."

"And he's mine," says Frank, though the fatigue in his voice seems to overwhelm him. "He'll be that forever. Excuse me," he says, "I've got to go check. His breathing hasn't been good. Excuse me."

"Good news and bad," says the Oncologist on Monday. He has knocked, entered the room, and now stands there. Their cots are unmade. One wastebasket is overflowing with coffee cups. "We've got the pathologist's report. The bad news is that the kidney they removed had certain lesions, called 'rests,' which are associated with a higher risk for disease in the other kidney. The good news is that the tumor is Stage I, regular cell structure, and under five hundred grams, which qualifies you for a national experiment in which chemotherapy isn't done but your boy is simply monitored with ultrasound. It's not all that risky, given that the patient's watched closely, but here is the literature on it. There are forms to sign, if you decide to do that. Read all this and we can discuss it further. You have to decide within four days."

Lesions? Rests? They dry up and scatter like M&M's on the floor. All she hears is the part about no chemo. Another sigh of relief rises up in her and spills out. In a life where there is only the bearable and the unbearable, a sigh of relief is an ecstasy.

"No chemo?" says the husband. "Do you recommend that?"

The Oncologist shrugs. What casual gestures these doctors are permitted! "I know chemo. I like chemo," says the Oncologist. "But this is for you to decide. It depends how you feel."

The Husband leans forward. "But don't you think that now that we have the upper hand with this thing we should keep going? Shouldn't we stomp on it, beat it, smash it to death with the chemo?"

The Mother swats him angrily and hard. "Honey, you're delirious!" She whispers, but it comes out as a hiss. "This is our lucky break!" Then she adds gently, "We don't want the Baby to have chemo."

The Husband turns back to the Oncologist. "What do you think?"

"It could be," he says, shrugging. "It could be that this is your lucky break. But you won't know for sure for five years."

The Husband turns back to the Mother. "O.K.," he says. "O.K."

The Baby grows happier and strong. He begins to move and sit and eat. Wednesday morning they are allowed to leave, and to leave without chemo. The Oncologist looks a little nervous. "Are you nervous about this?" asks the Mother.

"Of course I'm nervous." But he shrugs and doesn't look that nervous. "See you in six weeks for the ultrasound," he says, then he waves and leaves, looking at his big black shoes.

The Baby smiles, even toddles around a little, the sun bursting though the clouds, an angel chorus crescendoing. Nurses arrive. The Hickman is taken out of the Baby's neck and chest, antibiotic lotion is dispensed. The Mother packs up their bags. The baby sucks on a bottle of juice and does not cry.

"No chemo?" says one of the nurses. "Not even a little chemo?"

"We're doing watch-and-wait," says the Mother.

The other parents look envious but concerned. They have never seen any child get out of there with his hair and white blood cells intact.

"Will you be O.K.?" says Ned's mother.

"The worry's going to kill us," says the Husband.

"But if all we have to do is worry," chides the Mother, "every day for a hundred years, it'll be easy. It'll be nothing. I'll take all the worry in the world if it wards off the thing itself."

"That's right," says Ned's mother. "Compared to everything else, compared to all the actual events, the worry is nothing."

The Husband shakes his head. "I'm such an amateur," he moans.

"You're both doing admirably," says the other mother. "Your baby's lucky, and I wish you all the best."

The Husband shakes her hand warmly. "Thank you," he says. "You've been wonderful."

Another mother, the mother of Eric, comes up to them. "It's all very hard," she says, her head cocked to one side. "But there's a lot of collateral beauty along the way."

Collateral beauty? Who is entitled to such a thing? A child is ill. No one is entitled to any collateral beauty.

"Thank you," says the Husband.

Joey's father, Frank, comes up and embraces them both. "It's a journey," he says. He chucks the Baby on the chin. "Good luck, little man."

"Yes, thank you so much," says the Mother. "We hope things go well with Joey." She knows that Joey had a hard, terrible night.

Frank shrugs and steps back. "Gotta go," he says. "Goodbye!"

"Bye," she says, and then he is gone. She bites the inside of her lip, a bit tearily, then bends down to pick up the diaper bag, which is now stuffed with little animals; helium balloons are tied to its zipper. Shouldering the thing, the Mother feels she has just won a prize. All the parents have now vanished down the hall in the opposite direction. The Husband moves close. With one arm he takes the Baby from her; with the other he rubs her back. He can see she is starting to get weepy.

"Aren't these people nice? Don't you feel better hearing about their lives?" he asks.

Why does he do this, form clubs all the time—why does even this society of suffering soothe him? When it comes to death and dying, perhaps someone in this family ought to be more of a snob.

"All these nice people with their brave stories," he continues as they make their way toward the elevator bank, waving goodbye to the nursing staff as they go, even the Baby waving shyly. Bye-bye! Bye-bye! "Don't you feel consoled, knowing we're all in the same boat, that we're all in this together?"

But who on earth would want to be in this boat? the Mother thinks. This boat is a nightmare boat. Look where it goes: to a silver-and-white room, where, just before your eyesight and hearing and your ability to touch or be touched disappear entirely, you must watch your child die.

Rope! Bring on the rope.

"Let's make our own way," says the Mother, "and not in this boat."

Woman Overboard! She takes the Baby back from the Husband, cups the Baby's cheek in her hand, kisses his brow and then, quickly, his flowery mouth. The Baby's heart—she can hear it—drums with life. "For as long as I live," says the Mother, pressing the elevator button—up or down, everyone in the end has to leave this way—"I never want to see any of these people again."

There are the notes. Now, where is the money?

A Small, Good Thing

Raymond Carver

Saturday afternoon she drove to the bakery in the shopping center. After looking through a loose-leaf binder with photographs of cakes taped onto the pages, she ordered chocolate, the child's favorite. The cake she chose was decorated with a spaceship and launching pad under a sprinkling of white stars, and a planet made of red frosting at the other end. His name, SCOTTY, would be in green letters beneath the planet. The baker, who was an older man with a thick neck, listened without saying anything when she told him the child would be eight years old next Monday. The baker wore a white apron that looked like a smock. Straps cut under his arms, went around in back and then to the front again, where they were secured under his heavy waist. He wiped his hands on his apron as he listened to her. He kept his eyes down on the photographs and let her talk. He let her take her time. He'd just come to work and he'd be there all night, baking, and he was in no real hurry.

She gave the baker her name, Ann Weiss, and her telephone number. The cake would be ready on Monday morning, just out of the oven, in plenty of time for the child's party that afternoon. The baker was not jolly. There were no pleasantries between them, just the minimum exchange of words, the necessary information. He made her feel uncomfortable, and she didn't like that. While he was bent over the counter with the pencil in his hand, she studied his coarse features and wondered if he'd ever done anything else with his life besides be a baker. She was a mother and thirty-three years old, and it seemed to her that everyone, especially someone the baker's age—a man old enough to be her father—must have children who'd gone through this special time of cakes and birthday parties. There must be that between them, she thought. But he was abrupt with her—not rude, just abrupt. She gave up trying to make friends with him. She looked into the back of the bakery and could see a long, heavy wooden table with aluminum pie pans stacked at one end; and beside the table a metal container filled with empty racks. There was an enormous oven. A radio was playing country-western music.

The baker finished printing the information on the special order card and closed up the binder. He looked at her and said, "Monday morning." She thanked him and drove home.

On Monday morning, the birthday boy was walking to school with another boy. They were passing a bag of potato chips back and forth and the birthday boy was trying to find out what his friend intended to give him for his birthday that afternoon. Without looking, the birthday boy stepped off the curb at an intersection and was immediately knocked down by a car. He fell on his side with his head in the gutter and his legs out in the road. His eyes were closed, but his legs moved back and forth as if he were trying to climb over something. His friend dropped the potato chips and started to cry. The car had gone a hundred feet or so and stopped in the middle of the road. The man in the driver's seat looked back over his shoulder. He waited until the boy got unsteadily to his feet. The boy wobbled a little. He looked dazed, but okay. The driver put the car into gear and drove away.

The birthday boy didn't cry, but he didn't have anything to say about anything either. He wouldn't answer when his friend asked him what it felt like to be hit by a car. He walked home, and his friend went on to school. But after the birthday boy was inside his house and was telling his mother about it—she sitting beside him on the sofa, holding his hands in her lap, saying, "Scotty, honey, are you sure you feel all right, baby?" thinking she would call the doctor anyway—he suddenly lay back on the sofa, closed his eyes, and went limp. When she couldn't wake him up, she hurried to the telephone and called her husband at work. Howard told her to remain calm, remain calm, and then he called an ambulance for the child and left for the hospital himself.

Of course, the birthday party was canceled. The child was in the hospital with a mild concussion and suffering from shock. There'd been vomiting, and his lungs had taken in fluid which needed pumping out that afternoon. Now he simply seemed to be in a very deep sleep—but no coma, Dr. Francis had emphasized, no coma, when he saw the alarm in the parents' eyes. At eleven o'clock that night, when the boy seemed to be resting comfortably enough after the many X-rays and the lab work, and it was just a matter of his waking up and coming around, Howard left the hospital. He and Ann had been at the hospital with the child since that afternoon, and he was going home for a short while to bathe and change clothes. "I'll be back in an hour," he said. She nodded. "It's fine," she said. "I'll be right here." He kissed her on the forehead, and they touched hands. She sat in the chair beside the bed and looked at the child. She was waiting for him to wake up and be all right. Then she could begin to relax.

Howard drove home from the hospital. He took the wet, dark streets very fast, then caught himself and slowed down. Until now, his life had gone smoothly and to his satisfaction—college, marriage, another year of college for the advanced degree in business, a junior partnership in an investment firm. Fatherhood. He was happy and, so far, lucky—he knew that. His parents were still living, his brothers and his sister were established, his friends from college had gone out to take their places in the world. So far, he had kept away from any real harm, from those forces he knew existed and that could cripple or bring down a man if the luck went bad, if things suddenly turned. He pulled into the driveway and parked. His left leg began to tremble. He sat in the car for a minute and tried to deal with the present situation in a rational manner. Scotty had been hit by a car and was in the hospital, but he was going to be all right. Howard closed his eyes and ran his hand over his face. He got out of the car and went up to the front door. The dog was barking inside the house. The telephone rang and rang while he unlocked the door and fumbled for the light switch. He shouldn't have left the hospital, he shouldn't have. "Goddamn it!" he said. He picked up the receiver and said, "I just walked in the door!"

"There's a cake here that wasn't picked up," the voice on the other end of the line said.

"What are you saying?" Howard asked.

"A cake," the voice said. "A sixteen-dollar cake."

Howard held the receiver against his ear, trying to understand. "I don't know anything about a cake," he said. "Jesus, what are you talking about?"

"Don't hand me that," the voice said.

Howard hung up the telephone. He went into the kitchen and poured himself some whiskey. He called the hospital. But the child's condition remained the same; he was still sleeping and nothing had changed there. While water poured into the tub, Howard lathered his face and shaved. He'd just stretched out in the tub and closed his eyes when the telephone rang again. He hauled himself out, grabbed a towel, and hurried through the house, saying, "Stupid, stupid," for having left the hospital. But when he picked up the receiver and shouted, "Hello!" there was no sound at the other end of the line. Then the caller hung up.

He arrived back at the hospital a little after midnight. Ann still sat in the chair beside the bed. She looked up at Howard, and then she looked back at the child. The child's eyes stayed closed, the head was still wrapped in bandages. His breathing was quiet and regular. From an apparatus over the bed hung a bottle of glucose with a tube running from the bottle to the boy's arm.

"How is he?" Howard said. "What's all this?" waving at the glucose and the tube.

"Dr. Francis's orders," she said. "He needs nourishment. He needs to keep up his strength. Why doesn't he wake up, Howard? I don't understand, if he's all right."

Howard put his hand against the back of her head. He ran his fingers through her hair. "He's going to be all right. He'll wake up in a little while. Dr. Francis knows what's what."

After a time, he said, "Maybe you should go home and get some rest. I'll stay here. Just don't put up with this creep who keeps calling. Hang up right away."

"Who's calling?" she asked.

"I don't know who, just somebody with nothing better to do than call up people. You go on now."

She shook her head . "No," she said, "I'm fine."

"Really," he said. "Go home for a while, and then come back and spell me in the morning. It'll be all right. What did Dr. Francis say? He said Scotty's going to be all right. We don't have to worry. He's just sleeping now, that's all."

A nurse pushed the door open. She nodded at them as she went to the bedside. She took the left arm out from under the covers and put her fingers on the wrist, found the pulse, then consulted her watch. In a little while, she put the arm back under the covers and moved to the foot of the bed, where she wrote something on a clipboard attached to the bed.

"How is he?" Ann said. Howard's hand was a weight on her shoulder. She was aware of the pressure from his fingers.

"He's stable," the nurse said. Then she said, "Doctor will be in again shortly. Doctor's back in the hospital. He's making rounds right now."

"I was saying maybe she'd want to go home and get a little rest," Howard said. "After the doctor comes," he said.

"She could do that," the nurse said. "I think you should both feel free to do that, if you wish." The nurse was a big Scandinavian woman with blond hair. There was the trace of an accent in her speech.

"We'll see what the doctor says," Ann said. "I want to talk to the doctor. I don't think he should keep sleeping like this. I don't think that's a good sign." She brought her hand up to her eyes and let her head come forward a little. Howard's grip tightened on her shoulder, and then his hand moved up to her neck, where his fingers began to knead the muscles there.

"Dr. Francis will be here in a few minutes," the nurse said. Then she left the room.

Howard gazed at his son for a time, the small chest quietly rising and falling under the covers. For the first time since the terrible minutes after Ann's telephone call to him at his office, he felt a genuine fear starting in his limbs. He began shaking his head. Scotty was fine, but instead of sleeping at home in his own bed, he was in a hospital bed with bandages around his head and a tube in his arm. But this help was what he needed right now.

Dr. Francis came in and shook hands with Howard, though they'd just seen each other a few hours before. Ann got up from the chair. "Doctor?"

"Ann," he said and nodded. "Let's just first see how he's doing," the doctor said. He moved to the side of the bed and took the boy's pulse. He peeled back one eyelid and then the other. Howard and Ann stood beside the doctor and watched. Then the doctor turned back the covers and listened to the boy's heart and lungs with his stethoscope. He pressed his fingers here and there on the abdomen. When he was finished, he went to the end of the bed and studied the chart. He noted the time, scribbled something on the chart, and then looked at Howard and Ann.

"Doctor, how is he?" Howard said. "What's the matter with him exactly?"

"Why doesn't he wake up?" Ann said.

The doctor was a handsome, big-shouldered man with a tanned face. He wore a three-piece blue suit, a striped tie, and ivory cuff links. His gray hair was combed along the sides of his head, and he looked as if he had just come from a concert. "He's all right," the doctor said. "Nothing to shout about, he could be better, I think. But he's all right. Still, I wish he'd wake up. He should wake up pretty soon." The doctor looked at the boy again. "We'll know some more in a couple of hours, after the results of a few more tests are in. But he's all right, believe me, except for the hairline fracture of the skull. He does have that."

"Oh, no," Ann said.

"And a bit of a concussion, as I said before. Of course, you know he's in shock," the doctor said. "Sometimes you see this in shock cases. This sleeping."

"But he's out of any real danger?" Howard said. "You said before he's not in a coma. You wouldn't call this a coma, then—would you, doctor?" Howard waited. He looked at the doctor.

"No, I don't want to call it a coma," the doctor said and glanced over at the boy once more. 'He's just in a very deep sleep. It's a restorative measure the body is taking on its own. He's out of any real danger, I'd say that for certain, yes. But we'll know more when he wakes up and the other tests are in," the doctor said.

"It's a coma," Ann said. "Of sorts."

"It's not a coma yet, not exactly," the doctor said. "I wouldn't want to call it coma. Not yet, anyway. He's suffered shock. In shock cases, this kind of reaction is common enough; it's a temporary reaction to bodily trauma. Coma. Well, coma is a deep, prolonged unconsciousness, something that could go on for days, or weeks even. Scotty's not in that area, not as far as we can tell. I'm certain his condition will show improvement by morning. I'm betting that it will. We'll know more when he wakes up, which shouldn't be long now. Of course, you may do as you like, stay here or go home for a time. But by all means feel free to leave the hospital for a while if you want. This is not easy, I know." The doctor gazed at the boy again, watching him, and then he turned to Ann and said, "You try not to worry, little mother. Believe me, we re doing all that can be done. It's just a question of a little more time now." He nodded at her, shook hands with Howard again, and then he left the room.

Ann put her hand over the child's forehead. "At least he doesn't have a fever," she said. Then she said, "My God, he feels so cold, though. Howard? Is he supposed to feel like this? Feel his head."

Howard touched the child's temples. His own breathing had slowed. "I think he's supposed to feel this way right now," he said. "He's in shock, remember? That's what the doctor said. The doctor was just in here. He would have said something if Scotty wasn't okay."

Ann stood there a while longer, working her lip with her teeth. Then she moved over to her chair and sat down.

Howard sat in the chair next to her chair. They looked at each other. He wanted to say something else and reassure her, but he was afraid, too. He took her hand and put it in his lap, and this made him feel better, her hand being there. He picked up her hand and squeezed it. Then he just held her hand. They sat like that for a while, watching the boy and not talking. From time to time, he squeezed her hand. Finally, she took her hand away.

"I've been praying," she said.

He nodded.

She said, "I almost thought I'd forgotten how, but it came back to me. All I had to do was close my eyes and say, 'Please God, help us—help Scotty,' and then the rest was easy. The words were right there. Maybe if you prayed, too," she said to him.

"I've already prayed," he said. "I prayed this afternoon—yesterday afternoon, I mean—after you called, while I was driving to the hospital. I've been praying," he said.

"That's good," she said. For the first time, she felt they were together in it, this trouble. She realized with a start that, until now, it had only been happening to her and to Scotty. She hadn't let Howard into it, though he was there and needed all along. She felt glad to be his wife.

The same nurse came in and took the boy's pulse again and checked the flow from the bottle hanging above the bed.

In an hour, another doctor came in. He said his name was Parsons, from Radiology. He had a bushy moustache. He was wearing loafers, a western shirt, and a pair of jeans.

"We're going to take him downstairs for more pictures," he told them. "We need to do some more pictures, and we want to do a scan."

"What's that?" Ann said. "A scan?" She stood between this new doctor and the bed. "I thought you'd already taken all your X-rays."

"I'm afraid we need some more, he said. "Nothing to be alarmed about. We just need some more pictures, and we want to do a brain scan on him."

"My God," Ann said.

"It's perfectly normal procedure in cases like this," this new doctor said. "We just need to find out for sure why he isn't back awake yet. It's normal medical procedure, and nothing to be alarmed about. We'll be taking him down in a few minutes," this doctor said.

In a little while, two orderlies came into the room with a gurney. They were black-haired, dark-complexioned men in white uniforms, and they said a few words to each other in a foreign tongue as they unhooked the boy from the tube and moved him from his bed to the gurney. Then they wheeled him from the room. Howard and Ann got on the same elevator. Ann gazed at the child. She closed her eyes as the elevator began its descent. The orderlies stood at either end of the gurney without saying anything, though once one of the men made a comment to the other in their own language, and the other man nodded slowly in response.

Later that morning, just as the sun was beginning to lighten the windows in the waiting room outside the X-ray department, they brought the boy out and moved him back up to his room. Howard and Ann rode up on the elevator with him once more, and once more they took up their places beside the bed.

They waited all day, but still the boy did not wake up. Occasionally, one of them would leave the room to go downstairs to the cafeteria to drink coffee and then, as if suddenly remembering and feeling guilty, get up from the table and hurry back to the room. Dr. Francis came again that afternoon and examined the boy once more and then left after telling them he was coming along and could wake up at any minute now. Nurses, different nurses from the night before, came in from time to time. Then a young woman from the lab knocked and entered the room. She wore white slacks and a white blouse and carried a little tray of things which she put on the stand beside the bed. Without a word to them, she took blood from the boy's arm. Howard closed his eyes as the woman found the right place on the boy's arm and pushed the needle in.

"I don't understand this," Ann said to the woman.

"Doctor's orders," the young woman said. "I do what I'm told. They say draw that one, I draw. What's wrong with him, anyway?" she said. "He's a sweetie."

"He was hit by a car," Howard said. "A hit-and-run."

The young woman shook her head and looked again at the boy. Then she took her tray and left the room.

"Why won't he wake up?" Ann said. "Howard? I want some answers from these people."

Howard didn't say anything. He sat down again in the chair and crossed one leg over the other. He rubbed his face.He looked at his son and then he settled back in the chair, closed his eyes, and went to sleep.

Ann walked to the window and looked out at the parking lot. It was night, and cars were driving into and out of the parking lot with their lights on. She stood at the window with her hands gripping the sill, and knew in her heart that they were into something now, something hard. She was afraid, and her teeth began to chatter until she tightened her jaws. She saw a big car stop in front of the hospital and someone, a woman in a long coat, get into the car. She wished she were that woman and somebody, anybody, was driving her away from here to somewhere else, a place where she would find Scotty waiting for her when she stepped out of the car, ready to say Mom and let her gather him in her arms.

In a little while, Howard woke up. He looked at the boy again. Then he got up from the chair, stretched, and went over to stand beside her at the window. They both stared out at the parking lot. They didn't say anything. But they seemed to feel each other's insides now, as though the worry had made them transparent in a perfectly natural way.

The door opened and Dr. Francis came in. He was wearing a different suit and tie this time. His gray hair was combed along the sides of his head, and he looked as if he had just shaved. He went straight to the bed and examined the boy. "He ought to have come around by now. There's just no good reason for this," he said. "But I can tell you we're all convinced he's out of any danger. We'll just feel better when he wakes up. There's no reason, absolutely none, why he shouldn't come around. Very soon. Oh, he'll have himself a dilly of a headache when he does, you can count on that. But all of his signs are fine. They're as normal as can be."

"It is a coma, then?" Ann said.

The doctor rubbed his smooth cheek. "We'll call it that for the time being, until he wakes up. But you must be worn out. This is hard. I know this is hard. Feel free to go out for a bite," he said. "It would do you good. I'll put a nurse in here while you're gone if you'll feel better about going. Go and have yourselves something to eat."

"I couldn't eat anything," Ann said.

"Do what you need to do, of course," the doctor said. "Anyway, I wanted to tell you that all the signs are good, the tests are negative, nothing showed up at all, and just as soon as he wakes up he'll be over the hill."

"Thank you, doctor," Howard said. He shook hands with the doctor again. The doctor patted Howard's shoulder and went out.

"I suppose one of us should go home and check on things," Howard said. "Slug needs to be fed, for one thing."

"Call one of the neighbors," Ann said. "Call the Morgans. Anyone will feed a dog if you ask them to."

"All right," Howard said. After a while, he said, "Honey, why don't you do it? Why don't you go home and check on things, and then come back? It'll do you good. I'll be right here with him. Seriously," he said. "We need to keep up our strength on this. We'll want to be here for a while even after he wakes up.

"Why don't you go?" she said. "Feed Slug. Feed yourself."

"I already went," he said. "I was gone for exactly an hour and fifteen minutes. You go home for an hour and freshen up. Then come back."

She tried to think about it, but she was too tired. She closed her eyes and tried to think about it again. After a time, she said, "Maybe I will go home for a few minutes. Maybe if I'm not just sitting right here watching him every second, he'll wake up and be all right. You know? Maybe he'll wake up if I'm not here. I'll go home and take a bath and put on clean clothes. I'll feed Slug. Then I'll come back."

"I'll be right here," he said. "You go on home, honey. I'll keep an eye on things here." His eyes were bloodshot and small, as if he'd been drinking for a long time. His clothes were rumpled. His beard had come out again. She touched his face, and then she took her hand back. She understood he wanted to be by himself for a while, not have to talk or share his worry for a time. She picked her purse up from the nightstand, and he helped her into her coat.

"I won't be gone long," she said.

"Just sit and rest for a little while when you get home," he said. "Eat something. Take a bath. After you get out of the bath, just sit for a while and rest. It'll do you a world of good, you'll see. Then come back," he said. "Let's try not to worry. You heard what Dr. Francis said."

She stood in her coat for a minute trying to recall the doctor's exact words, looking for any nuances, any hint of something behind his words other than what he had said. She tried to remember if his expression had changed any when he bent over to examine the child. She remembered the way his features had composed themselves as he rolled back the child's eyelids and then listened to his breathing.

She went to the door, where she turned and looked back. She looked at the child, and then she looked at the father. Howard nodded. She stepped out of the room and pulled the door closed behind her.

She went past the nurses' station and down to the end of the corridor, looking for the elevator. At the end of the corridor, she turned to her right and entered a little waiting room where a Negro family sat in wicker chairs. There was a middle-aged man in a khaki shirt and pants, a baseball cap pushed back on his head. A large woman wearing a housedress and slippers was slumped in one of the chairs. A teenaged girl in jeans, hair done in dozens of little braids, lay stretched out in one of the chairs smoking a cigarette, her legs crossed at the ankles. The family swung their eyes to Ann as she entered the room. The little table was littered with hamburger wrappers and Styrofoam cups.

"Franklin," the large woman said as she roused herself. "Is it about Franklin?" Her eyes widened. "Tell me now, lady," the woman said. "Is it about Franklin?" She was trying to rise from her chair, but the man had closed his hand over her arm.

"Here, here," he said. "Evelyn."

"I'm sorry," Ann said. "I'm looking for the elevator. My son is in the hospital, and now I can't find the elevator."

"Elevator is down that way, turn left," the man said as he aimed a finger.

The girl drew on her cigarette and stared at Ann. Her eyes were narrowed to slits, and her broad lips parted slowly as she let the smoke escape. The Negro woman let her head fall on her shoulder and looked away from Ann, no longer interested.

"My son was hit by a car," Ann said to the man. She seemed to need to explain herself. "He has a concussion and a little skull fracture, but he's going to be all right. He's in shock now, but it might be some kind of coma, too. That's what really worries us, the coma part. I'm going out for a little while, but my husband is with him. Maybe he'll wake up while I'm gone."

"That's too bad," the man said and shifted in the chair. He shook his head. He looked down at the table, and then he looked back at Ann. She was still standing there. He said, "Our Franklin, he's on the operating table. Somebody cut him. Tried to kill him. There was a fight where he was at. At this party. They say he was just standing and watching. Not bothering nobody. But that don't mean nothing these days. Now he's on the operating table. We're just hoping and praying, that's all we can do now." He gazed at her steadily.

Ann looked at the girl again, who was still watching her, and at the older woman, who kept her head down, but whose eyes were now closed. Ann saw the lips moving silently, making words. She had an urge to ask what those words were. She wanted to talk more with these people who were in the same kind of waiting she was in. She was afraid, and they were afraid. They had that in common. She would have liked to have said something else about the accident, told them more about Scotty, that it had happened on the day of his birthday, Monday, and that he was still unconscious. Yet she didn't know how to begin. She stood looking at them without saying anything more.

She went down the corridor the man had indicated and found the elevator. She waited a minute in front of the closed doors, still wondering if she was doing the right thing. Then she put out her finger and touched the button.

She pulled into the driveway and cut the engine. She closed her eyes and leaned her head against the wheel for a minute. She listened to the ticking sounds the engine made as it began to cool. Then she got out of the car. She could hear the dog barking inside the house. She went to the front door, which was unlocked. She went inside and turned on lights and put on a kettle of water for tea. She opened some dog food and fed Slug on the back porch. The dog ate in hungry little smacks. It kept running into the kitchen to see that she was going to stay. As she sat down on the sofa with her tea, the telephone rang.

"Yes!" she said as she answered. "Hello!"

"Mrs. Weiss," a man's voice said. It was five o'clock in the morning, and she thought she could hear machinery or equipment of some kind in the background.

"Yes, yes! What is it?" she said. "This is Mrs. Weiss. This is she. What is it, please?" She listened to whatever it was in the background. "Is it Scotty, for Christ's sake?"

"Scotty," the man's voice said. "It's about Scotty, yes. It has to do with Scotty, that problem. Have you forgotten about Scotty?" the man said. Then he hung up.

She dialed the hospital's number and asked for the third floor. She demanded information about her son from the nurse who answered the telephone. Then she asked to speak to her husband. It was, she said, an emergency.

She waited, turning the telephone cord in her fingers. She closed her eyes and felt sick at her stomach. She would have to make herself eat. Slug came in from the back porch and lay down near her feet. He wagged his tail. She pulled at his ear while he licked her fingers. Howard was on the line.

"Somebody just called here," she said. She twisted the telephone cord. "He said it was about Scotty," she cried.

"Scotty's fine," Howard told her. "I mean, he's still sleeping. There's been no change. The nurse has been in twice since you've been gone. A nurse or else a doctor. He's all right."

"This man called. He said it was about Scotty," she told him.

"Honey, you rest for a little while, you need the rest. It must be that same caller I had. Just forget it. Come back down here after you've rested. Then we'll have breakfast or something."

"Breakfast," she said. "I don't want any breakfast."

"You know what I mean," he said. "Juice, something. I don't know. I don't know anything, Ann. Jesus, I'm not hungry, either. Ann, it's hard to talk now. I'm standing here at the desk. Dr. Francis is coming again at eight o'clock this morning. He's going to have something to tell us then, something more definite. That's what one of the nurses said. She didn't know any more than that. Ann? Honey, maybe we'll know something more then. At eight o'clock. Come back here before eight. Meanwhile, I'm right here and Scotty's all right. He's still the same," he added.

"I was drinking a cup of tea," she said, "when the telephone rang. They said it was about Scotty. There was a noise in the background. Was there a noise in the background on that call you had, Howard?"

"I don't remember," he said. "Maybe the driver of the car, maybe he's a psychopath and found out about Scotty somehow. But I'm here with him. Just rest like you were going to do. Take a bath and come back by seven or so, and we'll talk to the doctor together when he gets here. It's going to be all right, honey. I'm here, and there are doctors and nurses around. They say his condition is stable."

"I'm scared to death," she said.

She ran water, undressed, and got into the tub. She washed and dried quickly, not taking the time to wash her hair. She put on clean underwear, wool slacks, and a sweater. She went into the living room, where the dog looked up at her and let its tail thump once against the floor. It was just starting to get light outside when she went out to the car.

She drove into the parking lot of the hospital and found a space close to the front door. She felt she was in some obscure way responsible for what had happened to the child. She let her thoughts move to the Negro family. She remembered the name Franklin and the table that was covered with hamburger papers, and the teenaged girl staring at her as she drew on her cigarette. "Don't have children," she told the girl's image as she entered the front door of the hospital. "For God's sake, don't."

She took the elevator up to the third floor with two nurses who were just going on duty. It was Wednesday morning, a few minutes before seven. There was a page for a Dr. Madison as the elevator doors slid open on the third floor. She got off behind the nurses, who turned in the other direction and continued the conversation she had interrupted when she'd gotten into the elevator. She walked down the corridor to the little alcove where the Negro family had been waiting. They were gone now, but the chairs were scattered in such a way that it looked as if people had just jumped up from them the minute before. The tabletop was cluttered with the same cups and papers, the ashtray was filled with cigarette butts.

She stopped at the nurses' station. A nurse was standing behind the counter, brushing her hair and yawning.

"There was a Negro boy in surgery last night," Ann said. "Franklin was his name. His family was in the waiting room. I'd like to inquire about his condition."

A nurse who was sitting at a desk behind the counter looked up from a chart in front of her. The telephone buzzed and she picked up the receiver, but she kept her eyes on Ann.

"He passed away," said the nurse at the counter. The nurse held the hairbrush and kept looking at her. "Are you a friend of the family or what?"

"I met the family last night," Ann said. "My own son is in the hospital. I guess he's in shock. We don't know for sure what's wrong. I just wondered about Franklin, that's all. Thank you." She moved down the corridor. Elevator doors the same color as the walls slid open and a gaunt, bald man in white pants and white canvas shoes pulled a heavy cart off the elevator. She hadn't noticed these doors last night. The man wheeled the cart out into the corridor and stopped in front of the room nearest the elevator and consulted a clipboard. Then he reached down and slid a tray out of the cart. He rapped lightly on the door and entered the room. She could smell the unpleasant odors of warm food as she passed the cart. She hurried on without looking at any of the nurses and pushed open the door to the child's room.

Howard was standing at the window with his hands behind his back. He turned around as she came in.

"How is he?" she said. She went over to the bed. She dropped her purse on the floor beside the nightstand. It seemed to her she had been gone a long time. She touched the child's face. "Howard?"

"Dr. Francis was here a little while ago," Howard said. She looked at him closely and thought his shoulders were bunched a little.

"I thought he wasn't coming until eight o'clock this morning," she said quickly.

"There was another doctor with him. A neurologist."

"A neurologist," she said.

Howard nodded. His shoulders were bunching, she could see that. "What'd they say, Howard? For Christ's sake, what'd they say? What is it?"

"They said they're going to take him down and run more tests on him, Ann. They think they're going to operate, honey. Honey, they are going to operate. They can't figure out why he won't wake up. It's more than just shock or concussion, they know that much now. It's in his skull, the fracture, it has something, something to do with that, they think. So they're going to operate. I tried to call you, but I guess you'd already left the house."

"Oh, God," she said. "Oh, please, Howard, please," she said, taking his arms.

"Look!'" Howard said. "Scotty! Look, Ann!" He turned her toward the bed.

The boy had opened his eyes, then closed them. He opened them again now. The eyes stared straight ahead for a minute, then moved slowly in his head until they rested on Howard and Ann, then traveled away again.

"Scotty," his mother said, moving to the bed.

"Hey, Scott," his father said. "Hey, son."

They leaned over the bed. Howard took the child's hand in his hands and began to pat and squeeze the hand. Ann bent over the boy and kissed his forehead again and again. She put her hands on either side of his face. "Scotty, honey, it's Mommy and Daddy," she said. "Scotty?"

The boy looked at them, but without any sign of recognition. Then his mouth opened, his eyes scrunched closed, and he howled until he had no more air in his lungs. His face seemed to relax and soften then. His lips parted as his last breath was puffed through his throat and exhaled gently through the clenched teeth.

The doctors called it a hidden Occlusion and said it was a one-in-a-million circumstance. Maybe if it could have been detected somehow and surgery undertaken immediately, they could have saved him. But more than likely not. In any case, what would they have been looking for? Nothing had shown up in the tests or in the X-rays.

Dr. Francis was shaken. "I can't tell you how badly I feel. I'm so very sorry, I can't tell you," he said as he led them into the doctors' lounge. There was a doctor sitting in a chair with his legs hooked over the back of another chair, watching an early-morning TV show. He was wearing a green delivery room outfit, loose green pants and green blouse, and a green cap that covered his hair. He looked at Howard and Ann and then looked at Dr. Francis. He got to his feet and turned off the set and went out of the room. Dr. Francis guided Ann to the sofa, sat down beside her, and began to talk in a low, consoling voice. At one point, he leaned over and embraced her. She could feel his chest rising and falling evenly against her shoulder. She kept her eyes open and let him hold her. Howard went into the bathroom, but he left the door open. After a violent fit of weeping, he ran water and washed his face. Then he came out and sat down at the little table that held a telephone. He looked at the telephone as though deciding what to do first. He made some calls. After a time, Dr. Francis used the telephone.

"Is there anything else I can do for the moment?" he asked them.

Howard shook his head. Ann stared at Dr. Francis as if unable to comprehend his words.

The doctor walked them to the hospital's front door. People were entering and leaving the hospital. It was eleven o'clock in the morning. Ann was aware of how slowly, almost reluctantly, she moved her feet. It seemed to her that Dr. Francis was making them leave when she felt they should stay, when it would be more the right thing to do to stay. She gazed out into the parking lot and then turned around and looked back at the front of the hospital. She began shaking her head. "No, no," she said. "I can't leave him here, no." She heard herself say that and thought how unfair it was that the only words that came out were the sort of words used on TV shows where people were stunned by violent or sudden deaths. She wanted her words to be her own. "No," she said, and for some reason the memory of the Negro woman's head lolling on the woman's shoulder came to her. "No," she said again.

"I'll be talking to you later in the day," the doctor was saying to Howard. "There are still some things that have to be done, things that have to be cleared up to our satisfaction. Some things that need explaining."

"An autopsy," Howard said.

Dr. Francis nodded.

"I understand," Howard said. Then he said, "Oh, Jesus. No, I don't understand, doctor. I can't, I can't. I just can't."

Dr. Francis put his arm around Howard's shoulders. "I'm sorry. God, how I'm sorry." He let go of Howard's shoulders and held out his hand. Howard looked at the hand, and then he took it. Dr. Francis put his arms around Ann once more. He seemed full of some goodness she didn't understand. She let her head rest on his shoulder, but her eyes stayed open. She kept looking at the hospital. As they drove out of the parking lot, she looked back at the hospital.

At home, she sat on the sofa with her hands in her coat pockets. Howard closed the door to the child's room. He got the coffee-maker going and then he found an empty box. He had thought to pick up some of the child's things that were scattered around the living room. But instead he sat down beside her on the sofa, pushed the box to one side, and leaned forward, arms between his knees. He began to weep. She pulled his head over into her lap and patted his shoulder. "He's gone," she said. She kept patting his shoulder. Over his sobs, she could hear the coffee-maker hissing in the kitchen. "There, there," she said tenderly. "Howard, he's gone. He's gone and now we'll have to get used to that. To being alone."

In a little while, Howard got up and began moving aimlessly around the room with the box, not putting anything into it, but collecting some things together on the floor at one end of the sofa. She continued to sit with her hands in her coat pockets. Howard put the box down and brought coffee into the living room. Later, Ann made calls to relatives. After each call had been placed and the party had answered, Ann would blurt out a few words and cry for a minute. Then she would quietly explain, in a measured voice, what had happened and tell them about arrangements. Howard took the box out to the garage, where he saw the child's bicycle. He dropped the box and sat down on the pavement beside the bicycle. He took hold of the bicycle awkwardly so that it leaned against his chest. He held it, the rubber pedal sticking into his chest. He gave the wheel a turn.

Ann hung up the telephone after talking to her sister. She was looking up another number when the telephone rang. She picked it up on the first ring.

"Hello," she said, and she heard something in the background, a humming noise. "Hello!" she said. "For God's sake," she said. "Who is this? What is it you want?"

"Your Scotty, I got him ready for you," the man's voice said. "Did you forget him?"

"You evil bastard!" she shouted into the receiver. "How can you do this, you evil son of a bitch?"

"Scotty," the man said. "Have you forgotten about Scotty?" Then the man hung up on her.

Howard heard the shouting and came in to find her with her head on her arms over the table, weeping. He picked up the receiver and listened to the dial tone.

Much later, just before midnight, after they had dealt with many things, the telephone rang again.

"You answer it," she said. "Howard, it's him, I know." They were sitting at the kitchen table with coffee in front of them. Howard had a small glass of whiskey beside his cup. He answered on the third ring.

"Hello," he said. "Who is this? Hello! Hello!" The line went dead. "He hung up," Howard said. "Whoever it was."

"It was him," she said. "That bastard. I'd like to kill him," she said. "I'd like to shoot him and watch him kick," she said.

"Ann, my God," he said.

"Could you hear anything?" she said. "In the background? A noise, machinery, something humming?"

"Nothing, really. Nothing like that," he said. "There wasn't much time. I think there was some radio music. Yes, there was a radio going, that's all I could tell. I don't know what in God's name is going on," he said.

She shook her head. "If I could, could get my hands on him." It came to her then. She knew who it was. Scotty, the cake, the telephone number. She pushed the chair away from the table and got up. "Drive me down to the shopping center," she said. "Howard."

"What are you saying?"

"The shopping center. I know who it is who's calling. I know who it is. It's the baker, the son-of-a-bitching baker, Howard. I had him bake a cake for Scotty's birthday. That's who's calling. That's who has the number and keeps calling us. To harass us about that cake. The baker, that bastard."

They drove down to the shopping center. The sky was clear and stars were out. It was cold, and they ran the heater in the car. They parked in front of the bakery. All of the shops and stores were closed, but there were cars at the far end of the lot in front of the movie theater. The bakery windows were dark, but when they looked through the glass they could see a light in the back room and, now and then, a big man in an apron moving in and out of the white, even light. Through the glass, she could see the display cases and some little tables with chairs. She tried the door. She rapped on the glass. But if the baker heard them, he gave no sign. He didn't look in their direction.

They drove around behind the bakery and parked. They got out of the car. There was a lighted window too high up for them to see inside. A sign near the back door said THE PANTRY BAKERY, SPECIAL ORDERS. She could hear faintly a radio playing inside and something creak—an oven door as it was pulled down? She knocked on the door and waited. Then she knocked again, louder. The radio was turned down and there was a scraping sound now, the distinct sound of something, a drawer, being pulled open and then closed.

Someone unlocked the door and opened it. The baker stood in the light and peered out at them. "I'm closed for business," he said. "What do you want at this hour? It's midnight. Are you drunk or something?"

She stepped into the light that fell through the open door. He blinked his heavy eyelids as he recognized her. "It's you, he said.

"It's me," she said. "Scotty's mother. This is Scotty's father. We'd like to come in."

The baker said, "I'm busy now. I have work to do."

She had stepped inside the doorway anyway. Howard came in behind her. The baker moved back. "It smells like a bakery in here. Doesn't it smell like a bakery in here, Howard?"

"What do you want?" the baker said. "Maybe you want your cake? That's it, you decided you want your cake. You ordered a cake, didn't you?"

"You're pretty smart for a baker," she said. "Howard, this is the man who's been calling us." She clenched her fists. She stared at him fiercely. There was a deep burning inside her, an anger that made her feel larger than herself, larger than either of these men.

"Just a minute here," the baker said. "You want to pick up your three-day-old cake? That it? I don't want to argue with you, lady. There it sits over there, getting stale. I'll give it to you for half of what I quoted you. No. You want it? You can have it. It's no good to me, no good to anyone now. It cost me time and money to make that cake. If you want it, okay, if you don't, that's okay, too. I have to get back to work." He looked at them and rolled his tongue behind his teeth.

"More cakes," she said. She knew she was in control of it, of what was increasing in her. She was calm.

"Lady, I work sixteen hours a day in this place to earn a living," the baker said. He wiped his hands on his apron. "I work night and day in here, trying to make ends meet." A look crossed Ann's face that made the baker move back and say, "No trouble, now." He reached to the counter and picked up a rolling pin with his right hand and began to tap it against the palm of his other hand. "You want the cake or not? I have to get back to work. Bakers work at night," he said again. His eyes were small, mean-looking, she thought, nearly lost in the bristly flesh around his cheeks. His neck was thick with fat.

"I know bakers work at night," Ann said. "They make phone calls at night, too. You bastard," she said.

The baker continued to tap the rolling pin against his hand. He glanced at Howard. "Careful, careful," he said to Howard.

"My son's dead," she said with a cold, even finality. "He was hit by a car Monday morning. We've been waiting with him until he died. But, of course, you couldn't be expected to know that, could you? Bakers can't know everything—can they, Mr. Baker? But he's dead. He's dead, you bastard!" Just as suddenly as it had welled in her, the anger dwindled, gave way to something else, a dizzy feeling of nausea. She leaned against the wooden table that was sprinkled with flour, put her hands over her face, and began to cry, her shoulders rocking back and forth. "It isn't fair," she said. "It isn't, isn't fair."

Howard put his hand at the small of her back and looked at the baker. "Shame on you," Howard said to him. "Shame."

The baker put the rolling pin back on the counter. He undid his apron and threw it on the counter. He looked at them, and then he shook his head slowly. He pulled a chair out from under the card table that held papers and receipts, an adding machine, and a telephone directory. "Please sit down," he said. "Let me get you a chair," he said to Howard. "Sit down now, please." The baker went into the front of the shop and returned with two little wrought-iron chairs. "Please sit down, you people."

Ann wiped her eyes and looked at the baker. "I wanted to kill you," she said. "I wanted you dead."

The baker had cleared a space for them at the table. He shoved the adding machine to one side, along with the stacks of notepaper and receipts. He pushed the telephone directory onto the floor, where it landed with a thud. Howard and Ann sat down and pulled their chairs up to the table. The baker sat down, too.

"Let me say how sorry I am," the baker said, putting his elbows on the table. "God alone knows how sorry. Listen to me. I'm just a baker. I don't claim to be anything else. Maybe once, maybe years ago, I was a different kind of human being. I've forgotten, I don't know for sure. But I'm not any longer, if I ever was. Now I'm just a baker. That don't excuse my doing what I did, I know. But I'm deeply sorry. I'm sorry for your son, and sorry for my part in this," the baker said. He spread his hands out on the table and turned them over to reveal his palms. "I don't have any children myself, so I can only imagine what you must be feeling. All I can say to you now is that I'm sorry. Forgive me, if you can," the baker said. "I'm not an evil man, I don't think. Not evil, like you said on the phone. You got to understand what it comes down to is I don't know how to act anymore, it would seem. Please," the man said, "let me ask you if you can find it in your hearts to forgive me?"

It was warm inside the bakery. Howard stood up from the table and took off his coat. He helped Ann from her coat. The baker looked at them for a minute and then nodded and got up from the table. He went to the oven and turned off some switches. He found cups and poured coffee from an electric coffee-maker. He put a carton of cream on the table, and a bowl of sugar.

"You probably need to eat something," the baker said. "I hope you'll eat some of my hot rolls. You have to eat and keep going. Eating is a small, good thing in a time like this," he said.

He served them warm cinnamon rolls just out of the oven, the icing still runny. He put butter on the table and knives to spread the butter. Then the baker sat down at the table with them. He waited. He waited until they each took a roll from the platter and began to eat. "It's good to eat something," he said, watching them. "There's more. Eat up. Eat all you want. There's all the rolls in the world in here."

They ate rolls and drank coffee. Ann was suddenly hungry, and the rolls were warm and sweet. She ate three of them, which pleased the baker. Then he began to talk. They listened carefully. Although they were tired and in anguish, they listened to what the baker had to say. They nodded when the baker began to speak of loneliness, and of the sense of doubt and limitation that had come to him in his middle years. He told them what it was like to be childless all these years. To repeat the days with the ovens endlessly full and endlessly empty. The party food, the celebrations he'd worked over. Icing knuckle-deep. The tiny wedding couples stuck into cakes. Hundreds of them, no, thousands by now. Birthdays. Just imagine all those candles burning. He had a necessary trade. He was a baker. He was glad he wasn't a florist. It was better to be feeding people. This was a better smell anytime than flowers.

"Smell this," the baker said, breaking open a dark loaf.

"It's a heavy bread, but rich." They smelled it, then he had them taste it. It had the taste of molasses and coarse grains. They listened to him. They ate what they could. They swallowed the dark bread. It was like daylight under the fluorescent trays of light. They talked on into the early morning, the high, pale cast of light in the windows, and they did not think of leaving.

Strong Horse Tea

Alice Walker

Rannie Toomer's little baby boy Snooks was dying from double pneumonia and whooping cough. She sat away from him, gazing into the low fire, her long crusty bottom lip hanging. She was not married. Was not pretty. Was not anybody much. And he was all she had.

"Lawd, why don't that doctor come on here?" she moaned, tears sliding from her sticky eyes. She had not washed since Snooks took sick five days ago and a long row of whitish snail tracks laced her ashen face.

"What you ought to try is some of the old home remedies," Sarah urged. She was an old neighboring lady who wore magic leaves round her neck sewed up in possumskin next to a dried lizard's foot. She knew how magic came about, and could do magic herself, people said.

"We going to have us a doctor," Rannie Toomer said fiercely, walking over to shoo a fat winter fly from her child's forehead. "I don't believe in none of that swamp magic. All the old home remedies I took when I was a child come just short of killing me."

Snooks, under a pile of faded quilts, made a small gravelike mound in the bed. His head was like a ball of black putty wedged between the thin covers and the dingy yellow pillow. His little eyes were partly open, as if he were peeping out of his hard wasted skull at the chilly room, and the forceful pulse of his breathing caused a faint rustling in the sheets near his mouth like the wind pushing damp papers in a shallow ditch.

"What time you reckon that doctor'll git here?" asked Sarah, not expecting Rannie Toomer to answer her. She sat with her knees wide apart under many aprons and long dark skirts heavy with stains. From time to time she reached long cracked fingers down to sweep her damp skirts away from the live coals. It was almost spring, but the winter cold still clung to her bones and she had to almost sit in the fireplace to be warm. Her deep sharp eyes set in the rough leather of her face had aged a moist hesitant blue that gave her a quick dull stare like a hawk's. Now she gazed coolly at Rannie Toomer and rapped the hearthstones with her stick.

"White mailman, white doctor," she chanted skeptically, under her breath, as if to banish spirits.

"They gotta come see 'bout this baby," Rannie Toomer said wistfully. "Who'd go and ignore a little sick baby like my Snooks?"

"Some folks we don't know so well as we thinks we do might," the old lady replied. "What you want to give that boy of yours is one or two of the old home remedies; arrowsroot or sassyfras and cloves, or a sugar tit soaked in cat's blood."

Rannie Toomer's face went tight.

"We don't need none of your witch's remedies," she cried, grasping her baby by his shrouded toes, trying to knead life into him as she kneaded limberness into flour dough.

"We going to git some of them shots that makes peoples well, cures 'em of all they ails, cleans 'em out and makes 'em strong all at the same time."

She spoke upward from her son's feet as if he were an altar. "Doctor'll be here soon, baby," she whispered to him, then rose to look out the grimy window. "I done sent the mailman." She rubbed her face against the glass, her flat nose more flattened as she peered out into the rain.

"Howdy, Rannie Mae," the red-faced mailman had said pleasantly as he always did when she stood by the car waiting to ask him something. Usually she wanted to ask what certain circulars meant that showed pretty pictures of things she needed. Did the circulars mean that somebody was coming around later and would give her hats and suitcases and shoes and sweaters and rubbing alcohol and a heater for the house and a fur bonnet for her baby? Or, why did he always give her the pictures if she couldn't have what was in them? Or, what did the words say… especially the big word written in red: "S-A-L-E"?

He would explain shortly to her that the only way she could get the goods pictured on the circulars was to buy them in town and that town stores did their advertising by sending out pictures of their goods. She would listen with her mouth hanging open until he finished. Then she would exclaim in a dull amazed way that she never had any money and he could ask anybody. She couldn't ever buy any of the things in the pictures—so why did the stores keep sending them to her?

He tried to explain to her that everybody got the circulars, whether they had any money to buy with or not. That this was one of the laws of advertising and he could do nothing about it. He was sure she never understood what he tried to teach her about advertising, for one day she asked him for any extra circulars he had and when he asked what she wanted them for—since she couldn't afford to buy any of the items advertised—she said she needed them to paper the inside of her house to keep out the wind.

Today he thought she looked more ignorant than usual as she stuck her dripping head inside his car. He recoiled from her breath and gave little attention to what she was saying about her sick baby as he mopped up the water she dripped on the plastic door handle of the car.

"Well, never can keep 'em dry, I mean warm enough, in rainy weather like this here," he mumbled absently, stuffing a wad of circulars advertising hair driers and cold creams into her hands. He wished she would stand back from his car so he could get going. But she clung to the side gabbing away about "Snooks" and "NEWmonia" and "shots" and how she wanted a "REAL doctor."

"That right?" he injected sympathetically from time to time, and from time to time he sneezed, for she was letting in wetness and damp, and he felt he was coming down with a cold. Black people as black as Rannie Mae always made him uneasy, especially when they didn't smell good, and when you could tell they didn't right away. Rannie Mae, leaning in over him out of the rain, smelt like a wet goat. Her dark dirty eyes clinging to his face with such hungry desperation made him nervous.

Why did colored folks always want you to do something for them?

Now he cleared his throat and made a motion forward as if to roll up his window. "Well, ah, mighty sorry to hear 'bout that little fella," he said, groping for the window crank. "We'll see what we can do!" He gave her what he hoped was a big friendly smile. God! He didn't want to hurt her feelings! She looked so pitiful hanging there in the rain. Suddenly he had an idea.

"Whyn't you try some of old Aunt Sarah's home remedies?" he suggested brightly, still smiling. He half believed with everybody else in the county that the old blue-eyed black woman possessed magic. Magic that if it didn't work on whites probably would on blacks. But Rannie Mae almost turned the car over shaking her head and body with an empathic "NO!" She reached in a wet crusted hand to grasp his shoulder.

"We wants a doctor, a real doctor!" she screamed. She had begun to cry and drop her tears on him. "You git us a doctor from town," she bellowed, shaking the solid shoulder that bulged under his new tweed coat.

"Like I say," he drawled lamely although beginning to be furious with her, "we'll do what we can!" And he hurriedly rolled up the window and sped down the road, cringing from the thought that she had put her hands on him.

"Old home remedies! Old home remedies!" Rannie Toomer cursed the words while she licked at the hot tears that ran down her face, the only warmth about her. She turned back to the trail that led to her house, trampling the wet circulars under her feet. Under the fence she went and was in a pasture, surrounded by dozens of fat white folks' cows and an old gray horse and a mule or two. Animals lived there in the pasture all around her house, and she and Snooks lived in it.

It was less than an hour after she had talked to the mailman that she looked up expecting the doctor and saw old Sarah trampling through the grass on her walking stick. She couldn't pretend she wasn't home with the smoke climbing out the chimney, so she let her in, making her leave her bag of tricks on the front porch.

Old woman old as that ought to forgit trying to cure other people with her nigger magic…ought to use some of it on herself, she thought. She would not let her lay a finger on Snooks and warned her if she tried she would knock her over the head with her own cane.

"He coming, all right," Rannie Toomer said firmly, looking, straining her eyes to see through the rain.

"Let me tell you, child," the old woman said almost gently, "he ain't." She was sipping something hot from a dish. When would this one know, she wondered, that she could only depend on those who would come.

"But I told you," Rannie Toomer said in exasperation, as if explaining something to a backward child. "I asked the mailman to bring a doctor for my Snooks!"

Cold wind was shooting all around her from the cracks in the window framing, faded circulars blew inward from the walls. The old woman's gloomy prediction made her tremble.

"He done fetched the doctor," Sarah said, rubbing her dish with her hand. "What you reckon brung me over here in this here flood? Wasn't no desire to see no rainbows, I can tell you."

Rannie Toomer paled.

"I's the doctor, child." Sarah turned to Rannie with dull wise eyes. "That there mailman didn't git no further with that message than the road in front of my house. Lucky he got good lungs—deef as I is I had myself a time trying to make out what he was yellin'."

Rannie began to cry, moaning.

Suddenly the breathing of Snooks from the bed seemed to drown out the noise of the downpour outside. Rannie Toomer could feel his pulse making the whole house tremble.

"Here," she cried, snatching up the baby and handing him to Sarah. "Make him well. O my lawd, make him well!"

Sarah rose from her seat by the fire and took the tiny baby, already turning a purplish blue around the eyes and mouth.

"Let's not upset this little fella unnessarylike," she said, placing the baby back on the bed. Gently she began to examine him, all the while moaning and humming some thin pagan tune that pushed against the sound of the wind and rain with its own melancholy power. She stripped him of all his clothes, poked at his fibreless baby ribs, blew against his chest. Along his tiny flat back she ran her soft old fingers. The child hung on in deep rasping sleep, and his small glazed eyes neither opened fully nor fully closed.

Rannie Toomer swayed over the bed watching the old woman touching the baby. She thought of the time she had wasted waiting for the real doctor. Her feeling of guilt was a stone.

"I'll do anything you say do, Aunt Sarah," she cried, mopping at her nose with her dress. "Anything. Just, please God, make him git better!"

Old Sarah dressed the baby again and sat down in front of the fire. She stayed deep in thought for several moments. Rannie Toomer gazed first into her silent face and then at the baby, whose breathing seemed to have eased since Sarah picked him up.

Do something quick, she urged Sarah in her mind, wanting to believe in her powers completely. Do something that'll make him rise up and call his mama!

"The child's dying," said Sarah bluntly, staking out beforehand some limitation to her skill. "But there still might be something we can do…"

"What, Aunt Sarah, what?" Rannie Toomer was on her knees before the old woman's chair, wringing her hands and crying. She fastened hungry eyes on Sarah's lips.

"What can I do?" she urged fiercely, hearing the faint labored breathing from the bed.

"It's going to take a strong stomach," said Sarah slowly. "A mighty strong stomach. And most you young peoples these days don't have 'em."

"Snooks got a strong stomach," said Rannie Toomer, looking anxiously into the old serious face.

"It ain't him that's got to have the strong stomach," Sarah said, glancing down at Rannie Toomer. "You the one got to have a strong stomach…he won't know what it is he's drinking."

Rannie Toomer began to tremble way down deep in her stomach. It sure was weak, she thought. Trembling like that. But what could she mean her Snooks to drink? Not cat's blood—!" And not some of the messes with bat's wings she'd heard Sarah mixed for people sick in the head? …

"What is it?" she whispered, bringing her head close to Sarah's knee. Sarah leaned down and put her toothless mouth to her ear.

"The only thing that can save this child now is some good strong horse tea," she said, keeping her eyes on the girl's face. "The only thing. And if you wants him out of that bed you better make tracks to git some."

Rannie Toomer took up her wet coat and stepped across the porch into the pasture. The rain fell against her face with the force of small hailstones. She started walking in the direction of the trees where she could see the bulky lightish shapes of cows. Her thin plastic shoes were sucked at by the mud, but she pushed herself forward in search of the lone gray mare.

All the animals shifted ground and rolled big dark eyes at Rannie Toomer. She made as little noise as she could and leaned against a tree to wait.

Thunder rose from the side of the sky like tires of a big truck rumbling over rough dirt road. Then it stood a split second in the middle of the sky before it exploded like a giant firecracker, then rolled away again like an empty keg. Lightning streaked across the sky, setting the air white and charged.

Rannie Toomer stood dripping under her tree, hoping not to be struck. She kept her eyes carefully on the behind of the gray mare, who, after nearly an hour, began nonchalantly to spread her muddy knees.

At that moment Rannie Toomer realized that she had brought nothing to catch the precious tea in. Lightning struck something not far off and caused a crackling and groaning in the woods that frightened the animals away from their shelter. Rannie Toomer slipped down in the mud trying to take off one of her plastic shoes to catch the tea. And the gray mare, trickling some, broke for a clump of cedars yards away.

Rannie Toomer was close enough to catch the tea if she could keep up with the mare while she ran. So alternately holding her breath and gasping for air she started after her. Mud from her fall clung to her elbows and streaked her frizzy hair. Slipping and sliding in the mud she raced after the mare, holding out, as if for alms, her plastic shoe.

In the house Sarah sat, her shawls and sweaters tight around her, rubbing her knees and muttering under her breath. She heard the thunder, saw the lightning that lit up the dingy room and turned her waiting face to the bed. Hobbling over on stiff legs she could hear no sound; the frail breathing had stopped with the thunder, not to come again.

Across the mud-washed pasture Rannie Toomer stumbled, holding out her plastic shoe for the gray mare to fill. In spurts and splashes mixed with rainwater she gathered her tea. In parting, the old mare snorted and threw up one big leg, knocking her back into the mud. She rose, trembling and crying, holding the shoe, spilling none over the top but realizing a leak, a tiny crack at her shoe's front. Quickly she stuck her mouth there, over the crack, and ankle deep in the slippery mud of the pasture and freezing in her shabby wet coat, she ran home to give the still warm horse tea to her baby Snooks.

Indian Camp

Ernest Hemingway

At the lake shore there was another rowboat drawn up. The two Indians stood waiting.

Nick and his father got in the stern of the boat and the Indians shoved it off and one of them got in to row. Uncle George sat in the stern of the camp rowboat. The young Indian shoved the camp boat off and got in to row Uncle George.

The two boats started off in the dark. Nick heard the oarlocks of the other boat quite a way ahead of them in the mist. The Indians rowed with quick choppy strokes. Nick lay back with his father's arm around him. It was cold on the water. The Indian who was rowing them was working very hard, but the other boat moved further ahead in the mist all the time.

"Where are we going, Dad?" Nick asked.

"Over to the Indian camp. There is an Indian lady very sick."

"Oh," said Nick.

Across the bay they found the other boat beached. Uncle George was smoking a cigar in the dark. The young Indian pulled the boat way up on the beach. Uncle George gave both the Indians cigars.

They walked up from the beach through a meadow that was soaking wet with dew, following the young Indian who carried a lantern. Then they went into the woods and followed a trail that led to the logging road that ran back into the hills. It was much lighter on the logging road as the timber was cut away on both sides. The young Indian stopped and blew out his lantern and they all walked on along the road.

They came around a bend and a dog came out barking. Ahead were the lights of the shanties where the Indian bark-peelers lived. More dogs rushed out at them. The two Indians sent them back to the shanties. In the shanty nearest the road there was a light in the window. An old woman stood in the doorway holding a lamp.

Inside on a wooden bunk lay a young Indian woman. She had been trying to have her baby for two days. All the old women in the camp had been helping her. The men had moved off up the road to sit in the dark and smoke out of range of the noise she made. She screamed just as Nick and the two Indians followed his father and Uncle George into the shanty. She lay in the lower bunk, very big under a quilt. Her head was turned to one side. In the upper bunk was her husband. He had cut his foot very badly with an ax three days before. He was smoking a pipe. The room smelled very bad.

Nick's father ordered some water to be put on the stove, and while it was heating he spoke to Nick.

"This lady is going to have a baby, Nick," he said.

"I know," said Nick.

"You don't know," said his father. "Listen to me. What she is going through is called being in labor. The baby wants to be born and she wants it to be born. All her muscles are trying to get the baby born. That is what is happening when she screams."

"I see," Nick said.

Just then the woman cried out.

"Oh, Daddy, can't you give her something to make her stop screaming?" Nick asked.

"No. I haven't any anæsthetic," his father said. "But her screams are not important. I don't hear them because they are not important."

The husband in the upper bunk rolled over against the wall.

The woman in the kitchen motioned to the doctor that the water was hot. Nick's father went into the kitchen and poured about half of the water out of the big kettle into a basin. Into the water left in the kettle he put several things he unwrapped from a handkerchief.

"Those must boil," he said, and began to scrub his hands in the basin of hot water with a cake of soap he had brought from the camp. Nick watched his father's hands scrubbing each other with the soap. While his father washed his hands very carefully and thoroughly, he talked.

"You see, Nick, babies are supposed to be born head first but sometimes they're not. When they're not they make a lot of trouble for everybody. Maybe I'll have to operate on this lady. We'll know in a little while."

When he was satisfied with his hands he went in and went to work.

"Pull back that quilt, will you, George?" he said. "I'd rather not touch it."

Later when he started to operate Uncle George and three Indian men held the woman still. She bit Uncle George on the arm and Uncle George said, "Damn squaw bitch!" and the young Indian who had rowed Uncle George over laughed at him. Nick held the basin for his father. It all took a long time.

His father picked up the baby and slapped it to make it breathe and handed it to the old woman.

"See, it's a boy, Nick," he said. "How do you like being an interne?"

Nick said, "All right." He was looking away so as not to see what his father was doing.

"There. That gets it," said his father and put something into the basin.

Nick didn't look at it.

"Now," his father said, "there some stitches to put in. You can watch this or not, Nick, just as you like. I'm going to sew up the incision I made."

Nick did not watch. His curiosity had been gone for a long time.

His father finished and stood up. Uncle George and the three Indian men stood up. Nick put the basin out in the kitchen.

Uncle George looked at his arm. The young Indian smiled reminiscently.

"I'll put some peroxide on that, George," the doctor said.

He bent over the Indian woman. She was quiet now and her eyes were closed. She looked very pale. She did not know what had become of the baby or anything.

"I'll be back in the morning," the doctor said, standing up. "The nurse should be here from St. Ignace by noon and she'll bring everything we need."

He was feeling exalted and talkative as football players are in the dressing room after a game.

"That's one for the medical journal, George," he said. "Doing a Cæsarian with a jack-knife and sewing it up with nine-foot, tapered gut leaders."

Uncle George was standing against the wall, looking at his arm.

"Oh, you're a great man, all right," he said.

"Ought to have a look at the proud father. They're usually the worst sufferers in these little affairs," the doctor said. "I must say he took it all pretty quietly."

He pulled back the blanket from the Indian's head. His hand came away wet. He mounted on the edge of the lower bunk with the lamp in one hand and looked in. The Indian lay with his face toward the wall. His throat had been cut from ear to ear. The blood had flowed down into a pool where his body sagged the bunk. His head rested on his left arm. The open razor lay, edge up, in the blankets.

"Take Nick out of the shanty, George," the doctor said.

There was no need of that. Nick, standing in the door of the kitchen, had a good view of the upper bunk when his father, the lamp in one hand, tipped the Indian's head back.

It was just beginning to be daylight when they walked along the logging road back toward the lake.

"I'm terribly sorry I brought you along, Nickie," said his father, all his post-operative exhilaration gone. "It was an awful mess to put you through."

"Do ladies always have such a hard time having babies?" Nick asked.

"No, that was very, very exceptional."

"Why did he kill himself, Daddy?"

"I don't know, Nick. He couldn't stand things, I guess."

"Do many men kill themselves, Daddy?"

"Not very many, Nick."

"Do many women?"

"Hardly ever."

"Don't they ever?"

"Oh, yes. They do sometimes."

"Daddy?"

"Yes."

"Where did Uncle George go?"

"He'll turn up all right."

"Is dying hard, Daddy?"

"No, I think it's pretty easy, Nick. It all depends."

They were seated in the boat, Nick in the stern, his father rowing. The sun was coming up over the hills. A bass jumped, making a circle in the water. Nick trailed his hand in the water. It felt warm in the sharp chill of the morning.

In the early morning on the lake sitting in the stern of the boat with his father rowing, he felt quite sure that he would never die.

Bathtime
(*from* The Diving Bell and the Butterfly)

Jean-Dominique Bauby

At eight-thirty the physical therapist arrives. Brigitte, a woman with an athletic figure and an imperial Roman profile, has come to exercise my stiffened arms and legs. They call the exercise "mobilization," a term whose martial connotations contrast ludicrously with the paltry forces thus summoned, for I've lost sixty-six pounds in just twenty weeks. When I began a diet a week before my stroke, I never dreamed of such a dramatic result. As she works, Brigitte checks for the smallest flicker of improvement. "Try to squeeze my hand," she asks. Since I sometimes have the illusion that I am moving my fingers, I focus my energy on crushing her knuckles, but nothing stirs and she replaces my inert hand on its foam pad. In fact, the only sign of change is in my neck. I can now turn my head ninety degrees, and my field of vision extends from the slate roof of the building next door to the curious tongue-lolling Mickey Mouse drawn by my son, Theophile, when I was still unable to open my mouth. Now, after regular exercise, we have reached the stage of slipping a lollipop into it. As the neurologist says, "We need to be very patient." The session with Brigitte ends with a facial massage. Her warm fingers travel allover my face, including the numb zone, which seems to me to have the texture of parchment, and the area that still has feeling, where I can manage the beginnings of a frown. Since the demarcation line runs across my mouth, I can only half-smile, which fairly faithfully reflects my ups and downs. A domestic event as commonplace as washing can trigger the most varied emotions.

One day, for example, I can find it amusing, in my forty-fifth year, to be cleaned up and turned over, to have my bottom wiped and swaddled like a newborn's. I even derive a guilty pleasure from this total lapse into infancy. But the next day, the same procedure seems to me unbearably sad, and a tear rolls down through the lather a nurse's aide spreads over my cheeks. And my weekly bath plunges me simultaneously into distress and happiness. The delectable moment when I sink into the tub is quickly followed by nostalgia for the protracted immersions that were the joy of my previous life. Armed with a cup of tea or a Scotch, a good book or a pile of newspapers, I would soak for hours, maneuvering the taps with my toes. Rarely do I feel my condition so cruelly as when I am recalling such pleasures. Luckily I have no time for gloomy thoughts. Already they are wheeling me back, shivering, to my room, on a gurney as comfortable as a bed of nails. I must be fully dressed by ten-thirty and ready to go to the rehabilitation center. Having turned down the hideous jogging suit provided by the hospital, I am now attired as I was in my student days. Like the bath, my old clothes could easily bring back poignant, painful memories. But I see in the clothing a symbol of continuing life. And proof that I still want to be myself. If I must drool, I may as well drool on cashmere.

The Lost Mariner[1]

Oliver Sacks

You have to begin to lose your memory, if only in bits and pieces, to realise that memory is what makes our lives. Life without memory is no life at all ... Our memory is our coherence, our reason, our feeling, even our action. Without it, we are nothing ... (I can only wait for the final amnesia, the one that can erase an entire life, as it did my mother's ...) –Luis Buñuel

This moving and frightening segment in Buñuel's recently translated memoirs raises fundamental questions—clinical, practical, existential, philosophical: what sort of a life (if any), what sort of a world, what sort of a self, can be preserved in a man who has lost the greater part of his memory and, with this, his past, and his moorings in time?

It immediately made me think of a patient of mine in whom these questions are precisely exemplified: charming, intelligent, memoryless Jimmie G., who was admitted to our Home for the Aged near New York City early in 1975, with a cryptic transfer note saying, 'Helpless, demented, confused and disoriented.'

Jimmie was a fine-looking man, with a curly bush of grey hair, a healthy and handsome forty-nine-year-old. He was cheerful, friendly, and warm.

'Hiya, Doc!' he said. 'Nice morning! Do I take this chair here?' He was a genial soul, very ready to talk and to answer any questions I asked him. He told me his name and birth date, and the name of the little town in Connecticut where he was born. He described it in affectionate detail, even drew me a map. He spoke of the houses where his family had lived—he remembered their phone numbers still. He spoke of school and school days, the friends he'd had, and his special fondness for mathematics and science. He talked with enthusiasm of his days in the navy—he was seventeen, had just graduated from high school when he was drafted in 1943. With his good engineering mind he was a 'natural' for radio and electronics, and after a crash course in Texas found himself assistant radio operator on a submarine. He remembered the names of various submarines on which he had served, their missions, where they were stationed, the names of his shipmates. He remembered Morse code, and was still fluent in Morse tapping and touch-typing.

A full and interesting early life, remembered vividly, in detail, with affection. But there, for some reason, his reminiscences stopped. He recalled, and almost relived, his war days and service, the end of the war, and his thoughts for the future. He had come to love the navy, thought he might stay in it. But with the GI Bill, and support, he felt he might do best to go to college. His older brother was in accountancy school and engaged to a girl, a 'real beauty', from Oregon.

With recalling, reliving, Jimmie was full of animation; he did not seem to be speaking of the past but of the present, and I was very struck by the change of tense in his recollections as he passed from his school days to his days in the navy. He had been using the past tense, but now used the present—and (it seemed to me) not just the formal or fictitious present tense of recall, but the actual present tense of immediate experience.

A sudden, improbable suspicion seized me.

'What year is this, Mr G.?' I asked, concealing my perplexity under a casual manner.

'Forty-five, man. What do you mean?' He went on, We've won the war, FDR's dead, Truman's at the helm. There are great times ahead.'

'And you, Jimmie, how old would you be?'

Oddly, uncertainly, he hesitated a moment, as If engaged in calculation.

'Why, I guess I'm nineteen, Doc. I'll be twenty next birthday.'

Looking at the grey-haired man before me, I had an impulse for which I have never forgiven myself—it was, or would have been, the height of cruelty had there been any possibility of Jimmie's remembering it.

'Here,' I said, and thrust a mirror toward him. 'Look in the mirror and tell me what you see. Is that a nineteen-year-old looking out from the mirror?'

He suddenly turned ashen and gripped the sides of the chair. 'Jesus Christ,' he whispered. 'Christ, what's going on? What's happened to me? Is this a nightmare? Am I crazy? Is this a joke?'—and he became frantic, panicked.

'It's okay, Jimmie,' I said soothingly. 'It's just a mistake; nothing to worry about. Hey!' I took him to the window. 'Isn't this a lovely spring day. See the kids there playing baseball?' He regained his colour and started to smile, and I stole away, taking the hateful mirror with me.

Two minutes later I re-entered the room. Jimmie was still standing by the window, gazing with pleasure at the kids playing baseball below. He wheeled around as I opened the door, and his face assumed a cheery expression.

'Hiya, Doc!' he said. 'Nice morning! You want to talk to me—do I take this chair here?' There was no sign of recognition on his frank, open face.

'Haven't we met before, Mr G.?' I asked casually.

'No, I can't say we have. Quite a beard you got there. I wouldn't forget you, Doc!'

'Why do you call me "Doc"?'

'Well, you are a doc, ain't you?'

'Yes, but if you haven't met me, how do you know what I am?'

'You talk like a doc. I can see you're a doc.'

'Well, you're right, I am. I'm the neurologist here.'

'Neurologist? Hey, there's something wrong with my nerves? And "here"—where's "here"? What is this place anyhow?'

'I was just going to ask you—where do you think you are?'

'I see these beds, and these patients everywhere. Looks like a sort of hospital to me. But hell, what would I be doing in a hospital—and with all these old people, years older than me. I feel good, I'm strong as a bull. Maybe I work here ... Do I work? What's my job? ... No, you're shaking your head, I see in your eyes I don't work here. If I don't work here, I've been put here. Am I a patient, am I sick and don't know it, Doc? It's crazy, it's scary ... Is it some sort of joke?'

'You don't know what the matter is? You really don't know? You remember telling me about your childhood, growing up in Connecticut, working as a radio operator on submarines? And how your brother is engaged to a girl from Oregon?'

'Hey, you're right. But I didn't tell you that, I never met you before in my life. You must have read all about me in my chart.'

'Okay,' I said. 'I'll tell you a story. A man went to his doctor complaining of memory lapses. The doctor asked him some routine questions, and then said, "These lapses. What about them?" "What lapses?" the patient replied.'

'So that's my problem,' Jimmie laughed. 'I kinda thought it was. I do find myself forgetting things, once in a while—things that have just happened. The past is clear, though.'

'Will you allow me to examine you, to run over some tests?'

'Sure,' he said genially. 'Whatever you want.'

On intelligence testing he showed excellent ability. He was quick-witted, observant, and logical, and had no difficulty solving complex problems and puzzles—

no difficulty, that is, if they could be done quickly. If much time was required, he forgot what he was doing. He was quick and good at tic-tac-toe and checkers, and cunning and aggressive—he easily beat me. But he got lost at chess—the moves were too slow.

Honing in on his memory, I found an extreme and extraordinary loss of recent memory—so that whatever was said or shown to him was apt to be forgotten in a few seconds' time. Thus I laid out my watch, my tie, and my glasses on the desk, covered them, and asked him to remember these. Then, after a minute's chat, I asked him what I had put under the cover. He remembered none of them—or indeed that I had even asked him to remember. I repeated the test, this time getting him to write down the names of the three objects; again he forgot, and when I showed him the paper with his writing on it he was astounded, and said he had no recollection of writing anything down, though he acknowledged that it was his own writing, and then got a faint 'echo' of the fact that he had written them down.

He sometimes retained faint memories, some dim echo or sense of familiarity. Thus five minutes after I had played tic-tac-toe with him, he recollected that 'some doctor' had played this with him 'a while back'—whether the 'while back' was minutes or months ago he had no idea. He then paused and said, 'It could have been you?' When I said it was me, he seemed amused. This faint amusement and indifference were very characteristic, as were the involved cogitations to which he was driven by being so disoriented and lost in time. When I asked Jimmie the time of the year, he would immediately look around for some clue—I was careful to remove the calendar from my desk—and would work out the time of year, roughly, by looking through the window.

It was not, apparently, that he failed to register in memory, but that the memory traces were fugitive in the extreme, and were apt to be effaced within a minute, often less, especially if there were distracting or competing stimuli, while his intellectual and perceptual powers were preserved, and highly superior.

Jimmie's scientific knowledge was that of a bright high school graduate with a penchant for mathematics and science. He was superb at arithmetical (and also algebraic) calculations, but only if they could be done with lightning speed. If there were many steps, too much time, involved, he would forget where he was, and even the question. He knew the elements, compared them, and drew the periodic table—but omitted the transuranic elements.

'Is that complete?' I asked when he'd finished.

'It's complete and up-to-date, sir, as far as I know.'

'You wouldn't know any elements beyond uranium?'

'You kidding? There's ninety-two elements, and uranium's the last.'

I paused and flipped through a National Geographic on the table. 'Tell me the planets,' I said, 'and something about them.' Unhesitatingly, confidently, he gave me the planets—their names, their discovery, their distance from the sun, their estimated mass, character, and gravity.

'What's this?' I asked, showing him a photo in the magazine I was holding.

'It's the moon,' he replied.

'No, it's not,' I answered. 'It's a picture of the earth taken from the moon.'

'Doc, you're kidding! Someone would've had to get a camera up there!'

'Naturally.'

'Hell! You're joking—how the hell would you do that?'

Unless he was a consummate actor, a fraud simulating an astonishment he did not feel, this was an utterly convincing demonstration that he was still in the past. His words, his feelings, his innocent wonder, his struggle to make sense of what he saw, were precisely those of an intelligent young man in the forties faced with the future, with what had not yet happened, and what was scarcely imaginable. 'This more than anything else,' I wrote in my notes, 'persuades me that his cut-off around 1945 is genuine…What I showed him, and told him, produced the authentic amazement which it would have done in an intelligent young man of the pre-Sputnik era.'

I found another photo in the magazine and pushed it over to him.

'That's an aircraft carrier,' he said. 'Real ultramodern design. I never saw one quite like that.'

'What's it called?' I asked.

He glanced down, looked baffled, and said, 'The Nimitz!'

'Something the matter?'

'The hell there is!' he replied hotly. 'I know 'em all by name, and I don't know a Nimitz … Of course there's an Admiral Nimitz, but I never heard they named a carrier after him.'

Angrily he threw the magazine down.

He was becoming fatigued, and somewhat irritable and anxious, under the continuing pressure of anomaly and contradiction, and their fearful implications, to which he could not be entirely oblivious. I had already, unthinkingly, pushed him into panic, and felt it was time to end our session. We wandered over to the window again, and looked down at the sunlit baseball diamond; as he looked his face relaxed, he forgot the Nimitz, the satellite photo, the other horrors and hints, and became absorbed in the game below. Then, as a savoury smell drifted up from the dining room, he smacked his lips, said 'Lunch!', smiled, and took his leave.

And I myself was wrung with emotion—it was heartbreaking, it was absurd, it was deeply perplexing, to think of his life lost in limbo, dissolving.

'He is, as it were,' I wrote in my notes, 'isolated in a single moment of being, with a moat or lacuna of forgetting all round him ... He is man without a past (or future), stuck in a constantly changing, meaningless moment.' And then, more prosaically, 'The remainder of the neurological examination is entirely normal. Impression: probably Korsakov's syndrome, due to alcoholic degeneration of the mammillary bodies.' My note was a strange mixture of facts and observations, carefully noted and itemised, with irrepressible meditations on what such problems might 'mean', in regard to who and what and where this poor man was— whether, indeed, one could speak of an 'existence', given so absolute a privation of memory or continuity.

I kept wondering, in this and later notes—unscientifically—about 'a lost soul', and how one might establish some continuity, some roots, for he was a man without roots, or rooted only in the remote past.

'Only connect'—but how could he connect, and how could we help him to connect? What was life without connection? 'I may venture to affirm,' Hume wrote, 'that we are nothing but a bundle or collection of different sensations, which succeed each other with an inconceivable rapidity, and are in a perpetual flux and movement.' In some sense, he had been reduced to a 'Humean' being—I could not help thinking how fascinated Hume would have been at seeing in Jimmie his own philosophical 'chimaera' incarnate, a gruesome reduction of a man to mere disconnected, incoherent flux and change.

Perhaps I could find advice or help in the medical literature—a literature which, for some reason, was largely Russian, from Korsakov's original thesis (Moscow, 1887) about such cases of memory loss, which are still called 'Korsakov's syndrome', to Luria's Neuropsychology of Memory (which appeared in translation only a year after I first saw Jimmie). Korsakov wrote in 1887:

Memory of recent events is disturbed almost exclusively; recent impressions apparently disappear soonest, whereas impressions of long ago are recalled properly, so that the patient's ingenuity, his sharpness of wit, and his resourcefulness remain largely unaffected.

To Korsakov's brilliant but spare observations, almost a century of further research has been added—the richest and deepest, by far, being Luria's. And in Luria's account science became poetry, and the pathos of radical lostness was evoked. 'Gross disturbances of the organization of impressions of events and their sequence in time can always be observed in such patients,' he wrote. 'In consequence, they lose their integral experience of time and begin to live in a world of isolated impressions.' Further, as Luria noted, the eradication of impressions (and their disorder) might spread backward in time—'in the most serious cases—even to relatively distant events.'

Most of Luria's patients, as described in this book, had massive and serious cerebral tumours, which had the same effects as Korsakov's syndrome, but later spread and were often fatal. Luria included no cases of 'simple' Korsakov's syndrome, based on the self-limiting destruction that Korsakov described—neuron destruction, produced by alcohol, in the tiny but crucial mammillary bodies, the rest of the brain being perfectly preserved. And so there was no long-term follow-up of Luria's cases.

I had at first been deeply puzzled, and dubious, even suspicious, about the apparently sharp cut-off in 1945, a point, a date, which was also symbolically so sharp. I wrote in a subsequent note:

There is a great blank. We do not know what happened then—or subsequently ... We must fill in these 'missing' years—from his brother, or the navy, or hospitals he has been to ... Could it be that he sustained some massive trauma at this time, some massive cerebral or emotional trauma in combat, in the war, and that this may have affected him ever since? ... was the war his 'high point', the last time he was really alive, and existence since one long anti-climax?[2]

We did various tests on him (EEG, brain scans), and found no evidence of massive brain damage, although atrophy of the tiny mammillary bodies would not show up on such tests. We received reports from the navy indicating that he had remained in the navy until 1965, and that he was perfectly competent at that time.

Then we turned up a short nasty report from Bellevue Hospital, dated 1971, saying that he was 'totally disoriented ... with an advanced organic brain-syndrome, due to alcohol' (cirrhosis had also developed by this time). From Bellevue he was sent to a wretched dump in the Village, a so-called 'nursing home' whence he was rescued—lousy, starving—by our Home in 1975.

We located his brother, whom Jimmie always spoke of as being in accountancy school and engaged to a girl from Oregon. In fact he had married the girl from Oregon, had become a father and grandfather, and been a practising accountant for thirty years.

Where we had hoped for an abundance of information and feeling from his brother, we received a courteous but somewhat meagre letter. It was obvious from reading this—especially reading between the lines—that the brothers had scarcely seen each other since 1943, and gone separate ways, partly through the vicissitudes of location and profession, and partly through deep (though not estranging) differences of temperament. Jimmie, it seemed, had never 'settled down', was 'happy-go-lucky', and 'always a drinker'. The navy, his brother felt, provided a structure, a life, and the real problems started when he left it, in 1965. Without his habitual structure and anchor Jimmie had ceased to work, 'gone to pieces', and started to drink heavily. There had been some memory impairment, of the Korsakov type, in the middle and especially the late Sixties, but not so severe that Jimmie couldn't 'cope' in his nonchalant fashion. But his drinking grew heavier in 1970.

Around Christmas of that year, his brother understood, he had suddenly 'blown his top' and become deliriously excited and confused, and it was at this point he had been taken into Bellevue. During the next month, the excitement and delirium died down, but he was left with deep and bizarre memory lapses, or 'deficits,' to use the medical jargon. His brother had visited him at this time—they had not met for twenty years—and, to his horror, Jimmie not only failed to recognise him, but said, 'Stop joking! You're old enough to be my father. My brother's a young man, just going through accountancy school.'

When I received this information, I was more perplexed still: why did Jimmie not remember his later years in the navy, why did he not recall and organise his memories until 1970? I had not heard then that such patients might have a retrograde amnesia (see Postscript). 'I wonder, increasingly,' I wrote at this time, 'whether there is not an element of hysterical or fugal amnesia—whether he is not in flight from something too awful to recall', and I suggested he be seen by our psychiatrist. Her report was searching and detailed—the examination had included a sodium amytal test, calculated to 'release' any memories which might be repressed.

She also attempted to hypnotize Jimmie, in the hope of eliciting memories repressed by hysteria—this tends to work well in cases of hysterical amnesia. But it failed because Jimmie could not be hypnotized, not because of any 'resistance,' but because of his extreme amnesia, which caused him to lose track of what the hypnotist was saying. (Dr M. Homonoff, who worked on the amnesia ward at the Boston Veterans Administration hospital, tells me of similar experiences—and of his feeling that this is absolutely characteristic of patients with Korsakov's, as opposed to patients with hysterical amnesia.)

'I have no feeling or evidence,' the psychiatrist wrote, 'of any hysterical or "put-on" deficit. He lacks both the means and the motive to make a façade. His memory deficits are organic and permanent and incorrigible, though it is puzzling they should go back so long.' Since, she felt, he was 'unconcerned ... manifested no special anxiety ... constituted no management problem,' there was nothing she could offer, or any therapeutic 'entrance' or 'lever' she could see.

At this point, persuaded that this was, indeed, 'pure' Korsakov's, uncomplicated by other factors, emotional or organic, 1 wrote to Luria and asked his opinion. He spoke in his reply of his patient Bel,[3] whose amnesia had retroactively eradicated ten years. He said he saw no reason why such a retrograde amnesia should not thrust backward decades, or almost a whole lifetime. 'I can only wait for the final amnesia,' Buñuel writes, 'the one that can erase an entire life.' But Jimmie's amnesia, for whatever reason, had erased memory and time back to 1945—roughly— and then stopped. Occasionally, he would recall something much later, but the recall was fragmentary and dislocated in time. Once, seeing the word 'satellite' in a newspaper headline, he said offhandedly that he'd been involved in a project of satellite tracking while on the ship Chesapeake Bay, a memory fragment coming from the early or mid-Sixties. But, for all practical purposes, his cut-off point was during the mid- (or late) Forties, and anything subsequently retrieved was fragmentary, unconnected. This was the case in 1975, and it is still the case now, nine years later.

What could we do? What should we do? 'There are no prescriptions,' Luria wrote, 'in a case like this. Do whatever your ingenuity and your heart suggest. There is little or no hope of any recovery in his memory. But a man does not consist of memory alone. He has feeling, will, sensibilities, moral being—matters of which neuropsychology cannot speak. And it is here, beyond the realm of an impersonal psychology, that you may find ways to touch him, and change him. And the circumstances of your work especially allow this, for you work in a Home, which is like a little world, quite different from the clinics and institutions where I work. Neuropsychologically, there is little or nothing you can do; but in the realm of the Individual, there may be much you can do.'

Luria mentioned his patient Kur as manifesting a rare self-awareness, in which hopelessness was mixed with an odd equanimity. 'I have no memory of the present,' Kur would say. 'I do not know what I have just done or from where I have just come ... I can recall my past very well, but I have no memory of my present.' When asked whether he had ever seen the person testing him, he said, 'I cannot say yes or no, I can neither affirm nor deny that I have seen you.' This was sometimes the case with Jimmie; and, like Kur, who stayed many months in the same hospital, Jimmie began to form 'a sense of familiarity'; he slowly learned his way around the home—the whereabouts of the dining room, his own room, the elevators, the stairs, and in some sense recognised some of the staff, although he confused them, and perhaps had to do so, with people from the past. He soon became fond of the nursing sister in the Home; he recognised her voice, her footfalls, immediately, but would always say that she had been a fellow pupil at his high school, and was greatly surprised when I addressed her as 'Sister'.

'Gee!' he exclaimed, 'the damnedest things happen. I'd never have guessed you'd become a religious, Sister!'

Since he's been at our Home—that is, since early 1975—Jimmie has never been able to identify anyone in it consistently. The only person he truly recognises is his brother, whenever he visits from Oregon. These meetings are deeply emotional and moving to observe—the only truly emotional meetings Jimmie has. He loves his brother, he recognises him, but he cannot understand why he looks so old: 'Guess some people age fast,' he says. Actually his brother looks much younger than his age, and has the sort of face and build that change little with the years. These are true meetings, Jimmie's only connection of past and present, yet they do nothing to provide any sense of history or continuity. If anything they emphasise—at least to his brother, and to others who see them together—that Jimmie still lives, is fossilised, in the past.

All of us, at first, had high hopes of helping Jimmie—he was so personable, so likable, so quick and intelligent, it was difficult to believe that he might be beyond help. But none of us had ever encountered, even imagined, such a power of amnesia, the possibility of a pit into which everything, every experience, every event, would fathomlessly drop, a bottomless memory-hole that would engulf the whole world.

I suggested, when I first saw him, that he should keep a diary, and be encouraged to keep notes every day of his experiences, his feelings, thoughts, memories, reflections. These attempts were foiled, at first, by his continually losing the diary: it had to be attached to him—somehow. But this too failed to work: he dutifully kept a brief daily notebook but could not recognise his earlier entries in it. He does recognise his own writing, and style, and is always astounded to find that he wrote something the day before.

Astounded—and indifferent—for he was a man who, in effect, had no 'day before'. His entries remained unconnected and un-connecting and had no power to provide any sense of time or continuity. Moreover, they were trivial—'Eggs for breakfast', 'Watched ballgame on TV'—and never touched the depths. But were there depths in this unmemoried man, depths of an abiding feeling and thinking, or had he been reduced to a sort of Humean drivel, a mere succession of unrelated impressions and events?

Jimmie both was and wasn't aware of this deep, tragic loss in himself, loss of himself. (If a man has lost a leg or an eye, he knows he has lost a leg or an eye; but if he has lost a self—himself—he cannot know it, because he is no longer there to know it.) Therefore I could not question him intellectually about such matters.

He had originally professed bewilderment at finding himself amid patients, when, as he said, he himself didn't feel ill. But what, we wondered, did he feel? He was strongly built and fit, he had a sort of animal strength and energy, but also a strange inertia, passivity, and (as everyone remarked) 'unconcern'; he gave all of us an overwhelming sense of 'something missing', although this, if he realised it, was itself accepted with an odd 'unconcern'. One day I asked him not about his memory, or past, but about the simplest and most elemental feelings of all:

'How do you feel?'

'How do I feel,' he repeated, and scratched his head. 'I cannot say I feel ill. But I cannot say I feel well. I cannot say I feel anything at all.'

'Are you miserable?' I continued.

'Can't say I am.'

'Do you enjoy life?'

'I can't say I do ... '

I hesitated, fearing that I was going too far, that I might be stripping a man down to some hidden, unacknowledgeable, unbearable despair.

'You don't enjoy life,' I repeated, hesitating somewhat. 'How then do you feel about life?'

'I can't say that I feel anything at all.'

'You feel alive though?'

'Feel alive? Not really. I haven't felt alive for a very long time.'

His face wore a look of infinite sadness and resignation.

Later, having noted his aptitude for, and pleasure in, quick games and puzzles, and their power to 'hold' him, at least while they lasted, and to allow, for a while, a sense of companionship and competition—he had not complained of loneliness, but he looked so alone; he never expressed sadness, but he looked so sad—I suggested he be brought into our recreation programs at the Home. This worked better—better than the diary. He would become keenly and briefly involved in games, but soon they ceased to offer any challenge: he solved all the puzzles, and could solve them easily; and he was far better and sharper than anyone else at games. And as he found this out, he grew fretful and restless again, and wandered the corridors, uneasy and bored and with a sense of indignity—games and puzzles were for children, a diversion. Clearly, passionately, he wanted something to do: he wanted to do, to be, to feel—and could not; he wanted sense, he wanted purpose—in Freud's words, 'Work and Love'.

Could he do 'ordinary' work? He had 'gone to pieces', his brother said, when he ceased to work in 1965. He had two striking skills—Morse code and touch-typing. We could not use Morse, unless we invented a use; but good typing we could use, if he could recover his old skills—and this would be real work, not just a game. Jimmie soon did recover his old skill and came to type very quickly—he could not do it slowly—and found in this some of the challenge and satisfaction of a job. But still this was superficial tapping and typing; it was trivial, it did not reach to the depths. And what he typed, he typed mechanically—he could not hold the thought—the short sentences following one another in a meaningless order.

One tended to speak of him, instinctively, as a spiritual casualty—a 'lost soul': was it possible that he had really been 'de-souled' by a disease? 'Do you think he has a soul?' I once asked the Sisters. They were outraged by my question, but could see why I asked it. 'Watch Jimmie in chapel,' they said, 'and judge for yourself.'

I did, and I was moved, profoundly moved and impressed, because I saw here an intensity and steadiness of attention and concentration that I had never seen before in him or conceived him capable of. I watched him kneel and take the Sacrament on his tongue, and could not doubt the fullness and totality of Communion, the perfect alignment of his spirit with the spirit of the Mass. Fully, intensely, quietly, in the quietude of absolute concentration and attention, he entered and partook of the Holy Communion. He was wholly held, absorbed, by a feeling. There was no forgetting, no Korsakov's then, nor did it seem possible or imaginable that there should be; for he was no longer at the mercy of a faulty and fallible mechanism—that of meaningless sequences and memory traces—but was absorbed in an act, an act of his whole being, which carried feeling and meaning in an organic continuity and unity, a continuity and unity so seamless it could not permit any break.

Clearly Jimmie found himself, found continuity and reality, in the absoluteness of spiritual attention and act. The Sisters were right—he did find his soul here. And so was Luria, whose words now came back to me: 'A man does not consist of memory alone. He has feeling, will, sensibility, moral being ... It is here ... you may touch him, and see a profound change.' Memory, mental activity, mind alone, could not hold him; but moral attention and action could hold him completely.

But perhaps 'moral' was too narrow a word—for the aesthetic and dramatic were equally involved. Seeing Jim in the chapel opened my eyes to other realms where the soul is called on, and held, and stilled, in attention and communion. The same depth of absorption and attention was to be seen in relation to music and art: he had no difficulty, I noticed, 'following' music or simple dramas, for every moment in music and art refers to, contains, other moments. He liked gardening, and had taken over some of the work in our garden. At first he greeted the garden each day as new, but for some reason this had become more familiar to him than the inside of the Home. He almost never got lost or disoriented in the garden now; he patterned it, I think, on loved and remembered gardens from his youth in Connecticut.

Jimmie, who was so lost in extensional 'spatial' time, was perfectly organised in Bergsonian 'intentional' time; what was fugitive, unsustainable, as formal structure, was perfectly stable, perfectly held, as art or will. Moreover, there was something that endured and survived. If Jimmie was briefly 'held' by a task or puzzle or game or calculation, held in the purely mental challenge of these, he would fall apart as soon as they were done, into the abyss of his nothingness, his amnesia. But if he was held in emotional and spiritual attention—in the contemplation of nature or art, in listening to music, in taking part in the Mass in chapel—the attention, its 'mood', its quietude, would persist for a while, and there would be in him a pensiveness and peace we rarely, if ever, saw during the rest of his life at the Home.

I have known Jimmie now for nine years—and neuropsychologically, he has not changed in the least. He still has the severest, most devastating Korsakov's, cannot remember isolated items for more than a few seconds, and has a dense amnesia going back to 1945. But humanly, spiritually, he is at times a different man alto-gether—no longer fluttering, restless, bored, and lost, but deeply attentive to the beauty and soul of the world, rich in all the Kierkegaardian categories—and aes-thetic, the moral, the religious, the dramatic. I had wondered, when I first met him, if he was not condemned to a sort of 'Humean' froth, a meaningless flutter-ing on the surface of life, and whether there was any way of transcending the inco-herence of his Humean disease. Empirical science told me there was not—but empirical science, empiricism, takes no account of the soul, no account of what constitutes and determines personal being. Perhaps there is a philosophical as well as a clinical lesson here: that in Korsakov's, or dementia, or other such catastro-phes, however great the organic damage and Humean dissolution, there remains the undiminished possibility of reintegration by art, by communion, by touching the human spirit: and this can be preserved in what seems at first a hopeless state of neurological devastation.

Postscript

I know now that retrograde amnesia, to some degree, is very common, if not uni-versal, in cases of Korsakov's: The classical Korsakov's syndrome—a profound and permanent, but 'pure', devastation of memory caused by alcoholic destruction of the mammillary bodies—is rare, even among very heavy drinkers. One may, of course, see Korsakov's syndrome with other pathologies, as in Luria's patients with tumours. A particularly fascinating case of an acute (and mercifully transient) Korsakov's syndrome has been well described only very recently in the so-called Transient Global Amnesia (TGA) which may occur with migraines, head injuries or impaired blood supply to the brain. Here, for a few minutes or hours, a severe and singular amnesia may occur, even though the patient may continue to drive a car, or, perhaps, to carry on medical or editorial duties, in a mechanical way. But under this fluency lies a profound amnesia—every sentence uttered being forgot-ten as soon as it is said, everything forgotten within a few minutes of being seen, though long-established memories and routines may be perfectly preserved. (Some remarkable videotapes of patients during TGAs have recently [1986] been made by Dr John Hodges, of Oxford.)

Further, there may be a profound retrograde amnesia in such cases. My colleague Dr. Leon Protass tells me of a case seen by him recently, in which a highly intelli-gent man was unable for some hours to remember his wife or children, to remem-ber that he had a wife or children. In effect, he lost thirty years of his life—though, fortunately, for only a few hours. Recovery from such attacks is prompt and com-plete—yet they are, in a sense, the most horrifying of 'little strokes' in their power absolutely to annul or obliterate decades of richly lived, richly achieving, richly memoried life. The horror, typically, is only felt by others—the patient, unaware, amnesiac for his amnesia, may continue what he is doing, quite unconcerned, and only discover later that he lost not only a day (as is common with ordinary alcoholic 'blackouts'), but half a lifetime, and never knew it. The fact that one can lose the greater part of a lifetime has peculiar, uncanny horror.

In adulthood, life, higher life, may be brought to a premature end by strokes, senility, brain injuries, etc., but there usually re-mains the consciousness of life lived, of one's past. This is usually felt as a sort of compensation: 'At least I lived fully, tasting life to the full, before I was brain-injured, stricken, etc.' This sense of 'the life lived before', which may be either a consolation or a torment, is precisely what is taken away in retrograde amnesia. The 'final amnesia, the one that can erase an entire life' that Buñuel speaks of may occur, perhaps, in a terminal dementia, but not, in my experience, suddenly, in consequence of a stroke. But there is a different, yet comparable, sort of amnesia, which can occur suddenly—different in that it is not 'global' but 'modality—specific'.

Thus, in one patient under my care, a sudden thrombosis in the posterior circulation of the brain caused the immediate death of the visual parts of the brain. Forthwith this patient became completely blind—but did not know it. He looked blind—but he made no complaints. Questioning and testing showed, beyond doubt, that not only was he centrally or 'cortically' blind, but he had lost all visual images and memories, lost them totally—yet had no sense of any loss. Indeed, he had lost the very idea of seeing—and was not only unable to describe anything visually, but bewildered when I used words such as 'seeing' and 'light.' He had become, in essence, a non-visual being. His entire lifetime of seeing, of visuality, had, in effect, been stolen. His whole visual life had, indeed, been erased—and erased permanently in the instant of his stroke. Such a visual amnesia, and (so to speak) blindness to the blindness, amnesia for the amnesia, is in effect a 'total' Korsakov's, confined to visuality.

A still more limited, but none the less total, amnesia may be displayed with regard to particular forms of perception, as in the last chapter, 'The Man Who Mistook His Wife for a Hat'. There there was an absolute 'prosopagnosia', or agnosia for faces. This patient was not only unable to recognise faces, but unable to imagine or remember any faces—he had indeed lost the very idea of a 'face', as my more afflicted patient had lost the very ideas of 'seeing' or 'light.' Such syndromes were described by Anton in the 1890s. But the implication of these syndromes— Korsakov's and Anton's—what they entail and must entail for the world, the lives, the identities of affected patients, has been scarcely touched on even to this day.

In Jimmie's case, we had sometimes wondered how he might respond if taken back to his home town—in effect, to his pre-amnesia days—but the little town in Connecticut had become a booming city with the years. Later I did have occasion to find out what might happen in such circumstances, though this was with another patient with Korsakov's, Stephen R., who had become acutely ill in 1980 and whose retrograde amnesia went back only two years or so. With this patient, who also had severe seizures, spasticity and other problems necessitating in-patient care, rare weekend visits to his home revealed a poignant situation. In hospital he could recognise nobody and nothing, and was in an almost ceaseless frenzy of disorientation. But when his wife took him home, to his house which was in effect a 'time-capsule' of his pre-amnesia days, he felt instantly at home. He recognised everything, tapped the barometer, checked the thermostat, took his favourite armchair, as he used to do. He spoke of neighbours, shops, the local pub, a nearby cinema, as they had been in the mid-Seventies. He was distressed and puzzled if the smallest changes were made in the house. ('You changed the curtains today!' he once expostulated to his wife. 'How come? So suddenly? They were green this morning.' But they had not been green since 1978.) He recognised most of the neighbouring houses and shops—they had changed little between 1978 and 1983—but was bewildered by the 'replacement' of the cinema ('How could they tear it down and put up a supermarket overnight?'). He recognised friends and neighbours—but found them oddly older than he expected ('Old so-and-so! He's really showing his age. Never noticed it before. How come everyone's showing their age today?'). But the real poignancy, the horror, would occur when his wife brought him back—brought him, in a fantastic and unaccountable manner (so he felt), to a strange home he had never seen, full of strangers, and then left him. 'What are you doing?' he would scream, terrified and confused. What in the hell is this place? What the hell's going on?' These scenes were almost unbearable to watch, and must have seemed like madness, or nightmare, to the patient. Mercifully perhaps he would forget them within a couple of minutes.

Such patients, fossilised in the past, can only be at home, oriented, in the past. Time, for them, has come to a stop. I hear Stephen R. screaming with terror and confusion when he returns—screaming for a past which no longer exists. But what can we do? Can we create a time-capsule, a fiction? Never have I known a patient so confronted, so tormented, by anachronism, unless it was the 'Rose R.' of *Awakenings* (see 'Incontinent Nostalgia', Chapter Sixteen).

Jimmie has reached a sort of calm; William (Chapter Twelve) continually confabulates; but Stephen has a gaping time-wound, an agony that will never heal.

---

[1] After writing and publishing this history I embarked with Dr Elkhonon Goldberg—a pupil of Luria and editor of the original (Russian) edition of *The Neuropsychology of Memory*—on a close and systematic neuropsychological study of this patient. Dr Goldberg has presented some of the preliminary findings at conferences, and we hope in due course to publish a full account.

A deeply moving and extraordinary film about a patient with a profound amnesia (*Prisoner of Consciousness*), made by Dr Jonathan Miller, has just been shown in England (September 1986). A film has also been made (by Hilary Lawson) with a prosopagnosic patient (with many similarities to Dr P.). Such films are crucial to assist the imagination: 'What can be shown cannot be said.'

[2] In his fascinating oral history *The Good War* (1985) Studs Terkel transcribes countless stories of men and women, especially fighting men, who felt World War II was intensely real—by far the most real and significant time of their lives—everything since as pallid in comparison. Such men tend to dwell on the war and to relive its battles, comradeship, moral certainties and intensity. But this dwelling on the past and relative hebetude towards the present—this emotional dulling of current feeling and memory—is nothing like Jimmie's organic amnesia. I recently had occasion to discuss the question with Terkel: 'I've met thousands of men,' he told me, 'who feel they've just been "marking time" since '45—but I never met anyone for whom time terminated, like your amnesiac Jimmie.'

[3] See A.R. Luria, *The Neuropsychology of Memory* (1976), pp. 250-2.

Victories

For when the One Great Scorer comes
To write against your name,
He marks—not that you won or lost—
But how you played the game.

Grantland Rice

The Good Doctor

Susan Onthank Mates

Some years ago, during a winter that drove even the thieves and addicts indoors, Helen van Horne arrived to run the medicine department at City Hospital. Born in Wisconsin and just returned from Africa, she expected to feel at home in the South Bronx.

"Why," she asked Diana, as they rounded on the men's ward after a meeting of the community board, "do they hate me, so soon?"

"You look very clean," said Diana kindly, "your blouses are always white." She didn't add, you are so pale, your blue eyes so light they seem a disfigurement. Diana Figueroa was the medical chief resident for the year.

"Are you married?" asked Helen, noticing the gold band on Diana's smooth brown finger. "Yes," said Diana, and Helen imagined a home, two children, and a swing set. When Helen chose medical school, the act implied spinsterhood. Aware of her attractiveness, she tried but found herself unable to offer the standard plea for forgiveness: my patients, my students will be my children. Instead, she swept behind the parents who disapproved, the wedded college classmates, the condescending but lecherous professors, in the dust of her flight to Africa.

"What does your husband do?" she asked Diana.

"He said he wanted to be a lawyer." Diana finished writing in a chart, signed her name, and handed it to Helen.

"Oh," said Helen. "I suppose one of you might have to work part-time." She tried to imagine herself, when she was a young doctor, coming home at eight or nine in the evening, on her day off call, to talk to a child instead of throwing herself into bed.

"One of us does work part-time," said Diana. "When he works at all." She laughed. "Men," she said.

Helen began reading the chart. "I suppose that's fine, then," she said. She counter-signed Diana's note, which was incisive and succinct. I will help this chief resident, she thought. She is smart, like I was, and young enough to be my daughter. It pleased Helen to think of a daughter, married and a doctor.

In Tanzania, Helen ran a dispensary, single-handed, far into the bush. She operated by automobile headlight, diagnosed by her senses alone, tended the roses next to her well, and learned the language of solitude. "A good summer," she wrote to her sisters. "Not too much malaria, I've got the women to allow tetanus vaccination, now if only the generator doesn't break down again." She had two brief love affairs, otherwise the years passed from grassy summer to muddy winter to grassy summer like figures of a dance.

She slipped into relationship with the Masai and the earth: she cleaned the clinic each sunrise, ordered seasonal supplies with the solstice, and stopped numbering days entirely. She menstruated on the full moon, and the villagers came when they came, appearing unexpectedly on the horizon, carrying their sick in hammocks slung horizontally between tall men. After fifteen years, Helen described Tanzanian mountain fever in a clear and intelligent communication to the British journal *Lancet*, and because the virus was isolated from her specimens, and because it was interesting in its mode of replication and transmission, Helen's name became known.

On the day she received the letter from City Hospital, Helen folded it carefully into her skirt pocket, slung the rusted clinic shotgun on her back, and took the long path over the ridge. When she had first set up, the missionary nuns who preceded her said to always take the jeep. Lions, they warned earnestly, shaking their heads. Elephants. Rhinoceros.

Helen sat on a rock and watched a pair of gazelles leaping across the bleached grass on the other side of the ridge. In the distance, a giraffe swayed against the trees. I live in a garden of Eden, she thought, why would I ever want to leave? She looked down the way she had come, to the tin roof of her clinic. It was such an insignificant mark on the land, so easily removed. She traced the varicosities on her leg and felt suddenly afraid.

And so Diana became the guide of her return, pointing out the snow that bent the branches of the blue spruce whose roots cracked through the concrete of the long-abandoned formal entry to City Hospital. "I grew up on Willis Avenue," Diana told her, as they sat in the cafeteria.

"I grew up on a farm near Madison," Helen replied, "but my parents are dead. There's no one who knows me there now."

They sat for a moment, surveying the crowd of people, the yellowed linoleum, and the sturdy wooden tables. "Three types of students rotate here: do-gooders, voyeurs, and dropouts sent by the Dean," said Diana. She nodded down the table and Helen saw an extraordinarily beautiful young man with smooth, almost hairless golden skin, laughing and tossing his head. Like the African sun, thought Helen. Like sex.

"Mike Smith," said Diana. "A real goof-off. Kicked out everywhere else, the patients complained." Helen looked down at her lunch, conscious of her grey hair and how long it had been since she worked with men. She stared at the boiled tongue and sauerkraut.

"You'll get used to it," said Diana, "some cooks are Puerto Rican, some are from the South."

Helen took a bite of the meat. "I'll write a letter to the Dean," she said, "about that boy. These patients deserve consideration, too. A failing student should be failed."

"It won't," said Diana, "do any good."

Helen studied Diana's smooth face, her soft black eyebrows, and her neatly organized list of patients clipped to the board next to her lunch. "I hope you have enough time with your husband," said Helen. "I hope you decide to have children, soon, before you get too old."

In the afternoon of the day she came, Helen carried her two suitcases up to the staff quarters and sat on the narrow bed. There was a single bureau in the room, battered but solid oak, standing at a slight tilt on the warped linoleum. In the top drawer she found a tourniquet, a pen, index cards, and several unused needles. She picked them out carefully and dropped them into the garbage, then lined the drawer with paper towels from the sink. Folding her skirts into the bottom drawer, she found a package of condoms, tucked into the back right corner.

The window stuck several times before it finally creaked all the way up. Car horns, salsa music from the local bar, sirens, the sooty yearnings of urban life blasted into the room. Helen wrapped her arms around herself and stood, considering. She looked across at the decaying curve of the expressway, traffic crowded like wildebeest during mating season in the Serengeti. Then, turning back to the task of unpacking, she noticed faint fingernail scratches, hieroglyphics of passion, etched on the green wall at the head of the bed.

Over the next few months, Dr. Helen van Horne took charge of the department. She reviewed charts, observed procedures, met everyone including housekeepers and orderlies. "What disinfectant do you use?" she asked. "Why is this man waiting so long at X-ray?" She was on the wards at five in the morning and eleven at night, her faded hair pulled into a ponytail, starting an intravenous at a cardiac arrest, checking the diabetics' drawers for candy. Sometimes, standing in front of a wash-basin, or sitting at a deserted nursing station at the change of shift, she would sud-denly find herself watching the papery skin on the backs of her hands. What do I have to show for the years? she asked herself, but then a young woman gasping from rheumatic heart disease, or an old man bent with cancerous metastases passed by her, and she told herself: it doesn't matter. And she got back to work.

"What are they doing?" she asked Diana, as they passed a window looking toward the inner courtyard of the hospital. Michael Smith, the contours of his back glis-tening in the heat, kicked a ball toward some other students, boys and girls, who were encouraging several small children to kick it back.

"Oh," laughed Diana, "he's too much, isn't he?"

"The children will pull out their IVs," said Helen.

Diana walked around to the door. "Mr. Smith," she called, "the children will pull out their IV s."

"Anything you say Dr. Figueroa," said the boy.

"He played football for Harvard," said Diana, apologetically, when she came back inside.

"When you are a teacher," said Helen, looking back to check on the children but involuntarily glancing at Michael Smith's tight buttocks, "you must be careful about personal relationships. There is the issue of abuse of power." She looked away quickly, and with humiliation.

"Yes," said Diana. "But," she added, "the men do it all the time."

After that, Helen gave the teaching of the students over to Diana. She herself spent even more hours attending research meetings at the medical school and supervis-ing the medical service. She set up studies and chaired meetings. She read text-books of molecular biology. "We are beginning to see a new syndrome of infec-tions in IV drug users," she said in conference, and felt her power as the other doc-tors listened, because she was the Helen van Horne of Tanzanian mountain fever. She was senior and spoke with authority of microbial isolation and immune alter-ations. She submitted scholarly articles, and her roots spread into this identity, Chairman of Medicine at City Hospital. She stood taller, her walk grew firmer.

Once, she brought Diana with her to the medical school, to listen to her lecture. Afterwards, the men in the audience, who were division chiefs, but not depart-ment chairmen, spoke to her carefully and politely. The dean, who was the same age as Helen, came up to tease her about her theories, and Helen, who had, despite herself, imagined the touch of his hands and the feel of his skin, caught each barb and sent it back, leaning against the podium and laughing. But when she introduced Diana to him, he widened his stance. When Diana said how much she admired his research, he put his arm around her and introduced her to the other men, who, one after another, smiled with authority and watched her smooth brown cheeks.

Helen threw herself into work. "Examine these patients and report to me," she told the students. "Tell me if they are rude," she told the patients, "tell me if you think they will make good doctors," and the women always remarked on Michael Smith. Oh, they said, his hair, his eyes, his body. "He's careless," snapped Helen to Diana, "missed diagnoses, wrong medications." But when the boy stood to be rebuked, Helen felt the speculation in his eyes. She tightened her lips. "If you don't work, I will fail you, don't think I won't," she told him. But he glanced at her breasts and her nipples hardened.

"I don't want to be any super-doctor," he said, looking at her seriously. "I want to enjoy my life, you know what I mean?"

She laughed, because she had felt that way, too, then walked away. You are a fifty-year-old woman, she told herself. You are inappropriate. You are disgusting.

Later, on the wards, she rounded with Diana and set stern rules. "No more than six units of blood per bleeder," Helen said, after she watched an intern run ten units into a cirrhotic.

"But he's a young man," said Diana.

"He'll vomit up twice as much tomorrow," said Helen. "We don't have enough blood." She felt a pleasure in teaching this resident, after all the years of solitude. The girl would be a good doctor, she thought, but she needed disappointment.

"City Hospital," read the dean's reply, "has always been an albatross to the Medical School." It was spring now, and Helen watched the cornflowers pushing up through the cobbled ramp leading to the ambulance bay. She wondered if the dean had ever seen an albatross. Wingspan as wide as a man's arms, Daedalus, Icarus, she thought, and remembered the bird that followed them all the way from Dar es Salaam to Madagascar. Her lover was Indian, son of the supply ship's owner, a merchant in Oar. "Look," he said to her, as they were making love. His gold neckchain lay fallen in a spray of sweat from his dark chest onto hers, looped around one pink nipple. "You belong to me," he said. That was when her skin was smooth and firm, her hair a pale sheet of gold. She had wished, suddenly, and just for a moment, that a child, his child, would seed and grow in her womb. A year later, he was gone.

Helen fell into the rhythms of the Bronx. She met with Diana each morning and each evening. "The students," said Diana, "are improving."

"They need to be taught to do good," said Helen. "You are teaching them by example." She surprised herself. She had avoided a moral vocabulary. These had been the words of distance between herself and her parents: duty, family, obligation.

But Diana smiled and slicked back her hair. She had begun to wear it in a ponytail, too, a thick curly fall to complement Helen's thin fair one.

"Stick in the mud," Michael Smith teased her. "Dr. van Horne, Jr." He'd become friendly with the head of housekeeping, a middle-aged black man from Yonkers, and the two of them sat on the steps outside the emergency room talking football and joking, catcalling women as they walked by.

Diana stopped in front of him. "You left a patient in the hall last night and went off without signing him out. When I just happened to come by, he was already going into diabetic coma."

Michael Smith paled. "I'm sorry," he said.

"Tell it to the patient," said Diana, and left.

"But is he okay?" called Smith. She didn't answer.

Everyone in the hospital knew and respected Helen now. "Good morning, Doctor," she was greeted by the man who ladled out the scrambled eggs. "Good evening," by the woman mopping the women's ward. Sometimes the Spanish workers slipped and called her "Sister" when they stopped to thank her for taking care of a relative. Helen would glance at her own upright reflection in the glassed doors, curious to see how she might be mistaken for a nun.

She became convinced that this was how the people of the hospital saw her, as a nun, a medical missionary to the South Bronx. Bride of Christ, she taunted herself, standing in her room one night as the moonlight spread across the floor and crept up her ankles. Spinster Mother of City Hospital. How had this happened to her? That night she plaited her sheets into dreams: her nails became claws; her arms, wings of a nun's habit; and she felt the spring air rustle her belly as she swooped on a creature, garbage rat, skittering city mouse, swallowing its body with one snap while its head lay severed and bleeding on the ground.

Yes, she told herself, waking the next morning. The meaning of her years in Africa came to her suddenly as if in revelation. Apprenticeship. Learning to subjugate her will. She would dedicate herself to the patients and the students of City Hospital. Her face took on a pregnant glow, and she felt more content than she could remember in her life.

Because the dean would not remove Michael Smith, Helen decided she would make him into a doctor. She gave most of the teaching duties to Diana, but she no longer avoided the boy. To Diana she said, "You must think of how you will fit your practice around your family, and how you will choose a job where your husband can find work too." Diana smiled but said nothing. To Michael Smith, whom she caught leaving the hospital at five, with a blood sugar left unchecked, she said, "You must do whatever is necessary for the patients' good, even if it means you don't eat, don't sleep, or don't leave the hospital."

Smith flushed slightly, then looked over her left shoulder at a flurry of young nurses who were leaving, too, and said, "I'm going into radiology."

"Good," said Helen. "You'll make money. But first, you must pass your medicine rotation." As she walked away, she felt his eyes on the sway of her hips. Students, she told herself, become infatuated with the power of their teachers. Later that night, sitting at the bedside of a dying man, a drug addict infected on a hole he had eroded in his heart, Helen felt herself strengthen and harden in conviction. None of the private hospitals taught the concept of service. It was here the boy would learn to be a doctor, and it was her responsibility to teach him.

The third week of May began the wave of deaths. Death was of course a familiar presence at City Hospital, but like a wild tide, people began dying in unprecedented numbers. First, it was several cardiac failures on the men's wards, then a medication allergy on the women's ward, then one of the drug rehabilitation doctors fell out of a closet one morning, curled in the fetal position with a needle in his arm and stone-cold dead.

Helen called a meeting of the hospital's physicians. "I can't find a pattern," she said, "but I feel a connection, somewhere underneath." She didn't add, *and I feel somehow responsible.*

The next day *Staphylococcus* broke out in the neonatal nursery, crops of pustules erupted on even the heartiest of infants. Helen stood outside the plate glass of the babies' ward and watched the nurses wrap a tiny corpse, folding the blanket around the child, a flannel shroud. Why, she asked herself, because even Africa had not prepared her for the speed and the sweep of these deaths. Overcome, she paced the streets outside the hospital, walking blindly past the rubble, the garbage, and the deserted streets, in the long twilights of the late spring.

But the final straw was Henry, the chief of maintenance who sat, sighed, and fell over one day at dinner. It was Michael Smith who leapt on his chest and screamed, "Help," because he'd been sitting with Henry, once again, playing poker when he should have been drawing the evening bloods on the men's ward. They all came, residents, students, Helen, Diana. They ran a code in the cafeteria just as they would have in the emergency room: hooked up the EKG machine, pumped the chest, breathed in the slack mouth, started several large-bore IVs, and called to each other pulse, medication, paddles, step back, shock. But it was different, thought Helen, as she pierced the skin over his clavicle for a central line and glanced at his waxy face. It was Henry. She slipped and hit the artery. A geyser of blood sprayed her, Michael Smith, and the girl who was ventilating with the ambu-bag. When she got the vein, on the third try, she pushed it forward, but his blood clotted even as she pushed it in. "What the hell," she shouted, and there was a pause because they realized, inescapably, after fifteen minutes of flopping his flaccid blue arms, cracking his posthumous ribs, and watching the cardiogram read off an unremittingly straight line, that they were working on a dead man.

"Enough," said Helen. "Get a clean sheet. Wipe up this blood. Get these people out of here."

Michael Smith stood behind her, shaking and weeping, staring at Henry's still face. "His wife," he said, "his children."

"I'm sorry," said Helen.

The narrow hall that led to her room seemed longer than usual and peculiarly dry. She licked her lips, but her tongue stuck to the faint moisture on the roof of her mouth. She thought of calling Henry's wife, getting back to the wards, a memorial service, but the image of a corpse she had once found intruded. It was out in the bush at the end of the dry season, a young boy mauled by a lion so that one arm lay at an unnatural angle, connected only by a tendon that had hardened into rawhide. She stood at her door, looking straight ahead at the eroded slats.

The student, Michael Smith, came up behind her quietly. "Please," he said, touching her arm. She turned slowly and noticed that he was taller than she, how young he was, that his cheeks and nose were freckled with blood, and that he was still weeping.

"What do you want?" she asked him gently, but he just stared at her, moving his hand along her arm. "No," she said, seeing her pale face reflected in his eyes. He reached around her with his other arm and opened the door, pressing against her so she could feel the heat of his body radiating into her own. "Smith," she started, as he bent to kiss her neck. She felt revolted by her wave of desire, sick, like she might vomit. "Go away," she said, "now, before I have to report you to the dean." But when he looked up, his eyes wide and unfocused like a sleepwalker's, she pulled him to her breast and slowly licked the sweat that beaded across his face. "I'm sorry," she whispered. Afterwards, as he lay across her, naked and exhausted, she murmured it again, tracing his lips, "I'm sorry."

"I love you," Smith said, rolling over and going back to sleep, curling defenselessly. Helen stared at him, then got up and showered, letting the water run for hours down her face, between her legs. Then she chose her whitest blouse and went out onto the wards.

"Look," she said to the men's ward secretary. "Has the ward been repainted?"

"No," said the woman.

"But," Helen said in the nursery, "the babies are all so plump and healthy."

"Yes," said the practical nurse who was bathing a new arrival.

Helen walked a long path through the hospital. The women's ward had a new but familiar smell: dust soaked into earth, the beginning of the rainy season.

When she found Diana, she was going over cardiograms with Michael Smith in the emergency room.

"I called Henry's wife," said Diana.

"Yes," said Helen, taking the cardiogram from her, "what's wrong with this patient?"

"Thirty-year-old man with chest pain," began Diana, glancing over at Helen. Michael Smith was looking over Helen's shoulder at the strip of paper. Diana frowned. "Came in this morning," she went on. Michael ran his hand slowly up Helen's thigh. Diana stopped and stared at Helen, at her grey hair, at her grooved cheeks. Helen ex-amined the cardiogram as though nothing had happened.

Diana cleared her throat, her face mottled scarlet. "I understand, Dr. van Horne," she said, "that you've told Mr. Smith he will pass his medicine rotation?"

Helen didn't answer for a moment. "Will you take a fellowship next year?" she asked. "Of course, it is easier to adjust around a husband and children if you work in the emergency room."

"I left my husband," said Diana. "I wanted to be like you."

Helen looked down again at the cardiogram, but her hand began to shake. After a few minutes she said, "And do you think Mr. Smith should pass?"

"No," said Diana.

"Then fail him," said Helen.

"Christ," said Smith to Helen, "that's unfair." When she didn't answer, he looked wounded for a moment, then slammed out of the cubicle.

Diana stared at Helen, embarrassed. "He'll go to the dean," she started.

"Yes," said Helen, "he would be right to do that." She folded the cardiogram carefully back into the chart. She thought of Henry's dead body lying on the gurney waiting for his wife. His lips had turned a particular shade of blue, like the dusky sapphire of Lake Tanganyika at the last moment before the fall of night. It was the most beautiful color she had ever seen.

Helen sat on the bed in her room. "I regret to inform you," she wrote to the dean. She stopped and got up, staring at her face in the mirror, overcome with self-disgust. She seemed to herself grotesque, an old woman, a sexual vampire. "Is there ever any justification," she wrote on the wall beside the mirror, "for a teacher—" And yet, the deaths had stopped. She started again, "If A is a middle-aged woman, and B is a young male student, and insects grow, must grow in the rotted womb of fallen trees," but she lost interest and turned to the window. Cars honked and revved their engines, beasts of the Serengeti growled and spoke to her. She walked to the window and threw it open, as far as it would go. "It's the rainy season," she shouted to them, "order up the antibiotics, sow the crops." She saw them crowded on the expressway, antelope, giraffe, lions, surrounded by fields of ripened corn. "Yes," she whispered, because she felt at home. She heard the cry of the ambulances, the voices swelling from the emergency room, the beat of the hospital as it trembled with its load of humanity, and for her children, the patients and the students, she obeyed. She spread her arms Daedalus, Icarus, straight at the hot sun of the South Bronx, and hesitated.

Helen climbed down from the windowsill and sat at her desk. "The men," she said firmly, to herself, "do it all the time." She listened for a moment, for a rebuttal. Then she pulled on a white coat, to cover herself, and went out onto the wards.

Okay, So I'm in This Bed

Tony Gramaglia

Okay, so I'm in this bed. Hospital bed. Egg-crate cushion. Soft. Clean sheets. Inviting. I don't need to be in the bed, but I stay there. The TV keeps me there. The doctors keep me there. I keep me there. AIDS keeps me there. There are three chairs and even a sofa in the room, but I stay in the bed. My controls are there. Bed controls, TV controls. Nurse controls. Phone controls. Disease controls. I am the good patient in the bed. I can make doctors laugh. I can make nurses love me; I can welcome friends from this bed. This hospital bed.

At night I turn the TV on before I go to sleep. I put it on a nothing station that has only static and turn it up as loud as the remote will allow. I need the white noise to drown out the sound of AIDS. No people. I don't want to know that there are people. Down the hall. In that room next door or across the way. But the white noise of the TV still does not drown out the sounds of the hospital at night. The flushing of a toilet. That hacking cough. A pulling back of someone's curtain. A voice on the intercom. A faucet next door. My own breath.

You don't have to be awake to hear the screams of the man next door. You can't pretend it is just a sound. He is screaming, "No, no. Please don't. Please don't. Wait. Not now." And when the screaming stops and the coughing starts, I know they have stuck the tube down his throat to drain the fluid.

I know there are many scared eyes like mine opened now at 3:46 A.M. Eyes that are listening. There is a set in room 416. Another set in room 412. Another set of opened, scared eyes that should be shut and dreaming in room 411. But all of the eyes, those that can open if there is not too much morphine or Demerol in them, all those sets of eyes in the hospital beds are listening to this, to him. Or were.

You can close them now, your eyes. You wish you were someplace else so you could call the front desk and ask someone to please stop the man next door from dying so loudly. To stop injecting you with the fear of pain. To stop your eyes from listening to the death down the hall. In that room. In this room. In my room.

So close your eyes now. Listen to the white noise of the TV. Try to drown out the sounds. Drown out the fear. But the eyelids closed offer little peace. You can still see the empty room across the way where the black man used to be. You can't forget what you saw in another room, legs too skinny to be legs. You can see through the crack in the door the tangle of tubes that poke through another's chest. You can see her skin, too tight, too gray to be skin. You can see the fright.

At daybreak, I turn off the white noise. I am back in control. In this bed. I can make it go up or down. Call for a Coke. Turn a station. Open a blind. Flip on a light. Make a call. I keep feeling around for a switch to turn off the nights. Turn off the screams. Turn off the disease. But there is none. Not here. Not in this bed.

The Cowpath to America

Abraham Verghese

One night in 1979, toward the end of my interneship at the Government General Hospital in Madras, India, I was summoned from my bed to the contagious-diseases ward, where an elderly Brahman priest with rabies needed to be sedated. He was in one of two "dog bite" rooms: well-ventilated, high-ceilinged structures with no hard furniture, a padlocked door, and wire mesh on one wall. When I admitted him, two days previously, he had been lucid but had complained of fever and a tingling around the site of a healed bite wound. Now, as I stood, with the matron, peering into the cage, he was agitated and mumbling incoherently. I fished out a needle from the tabletop sterilizer and fitted it onto a syringe. I entered his room, squatted by his mat, gently rolled him to one side, and injected pethidine (Demerol) into his gluteus muscle. A plate of puri and potatoes lay untouched next to him; water had been taken away, because the sight of it gave him pharyngeal spasms.

I thought of my father's older brother, who was ten when he chased away a dog that had strayed into the compound of the family home in Kerala, South India. When the boy turned back to the house, the dog came up behind him and bit him on the hand. The wound was treated with a poultice by an Ayurvedic physician, but within a few weeks the child developed fever and confusion. The family knew what this meant. They made preparations to take him downriver by boat and from there by car to Trivandrum and the nearest big hospital. But the little boy screamed in terror at the sight of the river; it threw him into a fit of choking. Nothing could induce him to get on the boat. He died in the house where he was born.

The night matron ushered me out. "Cent per cent fatal, Doctor," she said as she locked the door after me. Then she added, "By morning? All over."

She would have laughed at my stupidity if I had told her that, according to "Harrison's Principles of Internal Medicine," my American textbook, a rabid patient could survive. One patient, the book said, had been maintained for months on a respirator, in a state-of-the-art intensive-care unit, until the virus burned itself out. But then in America only a few human rabies cases occurred every year. Around twenty-five thousand people died of rabies annually in India. Our intensive-care beds were needed for people who had better chances of survival.

I walked back to my quarters, through a maze of walkways that led past the open wards. When I first entered the hospital, as a third-year medical student, the redolence of the wards had been exciting—a vindication for the years of sitting through dry lectures on anatomy, biochemistry, and physiology. My hero was Professor K. V. Thiruvengadam. During my first day on the wards, as fifteen of us students trooped behind him on rounds, we came to a patient giving off a strange smell, and it seemed to animate Professor K.V.T. He rattled off a litany of odors— the acetone breath of diabetic coma, the freshly-baked-bread odor of typhoid fever, the stale-beer stench of scrofula, the sewer breath of a lung abscess, the just-plucked-chicken-feathers emanation of rubella—before ar-riving at the ammoniacal, mousy odor that rose from the patient before us. "Hepatic coma," he said, and he proceeded to demonstrate all its other signs.

K.V.T. could percuss a lung and predict precisely what the chest X-ray would look like. He would quote Thackeray, Nature, and the most recent edition of "Harrison's." As chief of medicine, he was a busy man, but he made us feel that there was nothing more important to him than guiding our fingers to feel what he felt, and guiding our eyes and ears to see and hear what he saw and heard.

But three years after I met him—half-way through my compulsory internship— my excitement had worn off. It had given way to a sense of impotence. Oh, yes, our hospital performed open-heart surgery; we had a giant neurosurgical institute; and we provided yeoman service in many other areas. But the demands always outstripped the resources. In the lines that wove and doubled back on themselves at the door of the outpatient clinic each morning, almost every patient would have been deserving of hospital admission by American standards. But only some were picked for admission, and then often because the patient was a good "teaching case." At exam time, professional patients would come to the hospital and receive a week's lodging and food in return for being fodder for the examinees. Takedown Govindraj, for instance, would, if you got him as your assigned case, signal to you to get your pen out. (A few rupees would have had to pass between examinee and patient before this step.) "Take down, Doctor," he'd say, adopting the tone of the many clinicians who had used his body to instruct medical students. "Take down: jaundice, spider angiomas, palmar erythema, Dupuytren's contracture, flapping tremor, breast enlargement, splenomegaly, shrunken liver, testicular atrophy." He would point to each of the stigmata of cirrhosis and pronounce the words pretty well, considering that he spoke no English. But it was best for the examinee to know this stuff on his own. Takedown occasionally sent out for mutton biriyani, which was more protein than his liver could handle. The mild hepatic encephalopathy that resulted would cause him to say "breast enlargement" while pointing to his balls.

The corridor outside the operating rooms was now dark and silent. The daytime cacophony of auto rickshaws, scooters, mopeds, cars, and buses outside the hospital walls and the crush of people within had lessened. The white-washed pillars that held up the buildings were faintly visible. It was possible, in the dim glow of the metal-caged light bulbs, to ignore the betel-juice stains and to imagine the colonial era, when British medical officers had ruled like emperors here and had trained "native" medical students, teaching them about Pott's disease and Hansen's disease and Sydenham's chorea and other white-male-eponym conditions, and instilling in them the desire to wear pith helmets and white cotton suits and own Raleigh bicycles and, one day, sail to England and bring home a cherished F.R.C.P. (Fellow of the Royal College of Physicians) or F.R.C.S. (Fellow of the Royal College of Surgeons).

Once again, I calculated how many days of my interneship I had left before I could leave India. I was twenty-five and restless and I had decided to pursue specialty training in America. I had been educated in India for the most part, but was born in Ethiopia, where my expatriate-Indian parents were teachers. By the time I reached medical school, my parents had emigrated to America. My older brother had finished engineering school in Madras and was now at M.I.T., in Cambridge. My parents had filed all the necessary papers, and I had a green card. The door was open for me to leave.

Most of my friends in India had, like me, grown up speaking English in the house, thinking in English, reading first Enid Blyton's Famous Five books and then the Hardy Boys. Increasingly, by the late seventies, it seemed as if we merely had our physical existence in India; mentally, we lived in a fantasy world that was somehow removed from the dust and the traffic and the chaos outside. It often appeared to me that my friends' parents and grandparents were doing the same thing we were. Their escape was the world of "the old days," by which, strangely, they meant the British days and the era of the maharajas and princely states and the rituals of afternoon tea. Our escape was the America of "Woodstock," the documentary (which, like most things, came to India years after the actual event, but seemed to trigger its own revolution among the already Westernized kids I knew). For us, America was defined by the music of Crosby, Stills, Nash and Young and by the novels of John Irving and Joseph Heller. Our preference for America was also a form of rebellion against the British fixation of our elders. England seemed to be a dead-end place, particularly for a young medical student. You could get your

F.R.C.S. (Farting Round the Countryside, we called it), but you would almost never be appointed a consultant. You either stayed as a perpetual interne or took your precious F.R.C.S. back to Madras and hung up your shingle and competed with all the other " 'phoren' returned" doctors on Sterling Road.

Those of us who planned to get to America abandoned British and Indian texts, which tended to be dogmatic, imperious tomes. "Harrison's" had numerous authors, and it quoted the pivotal, and even controversial, studies—the Tuskegee study of untreated syphilis, for example—that formed the basis of modern practice. I would pick out names from the seven-page list of contributors to the seventh edition and read them aloud, enjoying the way the elegant titles rolled off my tongue and fantasizing about one day being the Hersey Professor of the Theory and Practice of Physic (Medicine), Harvard Medical School.

It was possible to get an internship as a foreign medical graduate (F.M.G.) in America. Residency programs in many inner-city American hospitals needed foreign medical graduates, and recruited them vigorously. These were institutions that rarely attracted American medical school graduates. The hospitals' residency programs were supported by Medicare educational money, and they served an indigent patient population. The annual influx of foreign medical graduates was vital to the hospitals' functioning.

Yet while it was possible to get an American interneship, it wasn't easy. First, you had to pass a daylong examination that tested your medical knowledge, and another that tested your proficiency in English. By the end of the sixties, the exam was no longer offered in India. The closest places where the exam could be taken ended up being in Thailand, the Philippines, and Singapore. It seemed to us that, through the seventies and eighties, the bar kept being raised; the exam became more specialized, with the two parts given at different times of the year. Undaunted, medical students, their heads buried in study guides, packed the twice-a-year charter planes that took off from Madras or Bombay. Fewer than fifty per cent of the students passed the exams; a larger percentage probably lost their virginity in Bangkok or Manila.

The biggest hurdle, though, came after the exams, with the attempt to get a visa from the American Consulate. In the late seventies, it was exceedingly difficult for an Indian doctor to obtain a visa to go to America. But this didn't stop people who had passed the exams from trying. The main visa officer was a black gentleman who, rumor had it, hated his posting. The lines outside the Consulate would form the night before. Most people were dressed in their consulate best, but some scruffy-looking touts wearing sarongs squatted in line all night and made a good living selling their spots to late arrivals. For a fee, a pundit whose credentials were dubious—after all, if he knew how to get a visa, what was he doing in Madras?—would coach you on how to be "cent per cent successful."

From the sweltering humidity outdoors I entered the spotless, air-conditioned antechamber of the Consulate, with its United States flag, its orange carpets, and its photograph of Jimmy Carter. My visit was routine, since I had a green card. But my classmates who were applying for tourist visas or work visas needed an "interview" to prove that they planned to return to India. They carried with them surety bonds, land certificates, bank statements, and anything else that signified wealth in India, as proof that they were not going to America to better themselves—they were doing just fabulously in India, thank you very much. Relatives often transferred all their assets to an applicant for twenty-four hours, so that the applicant could be rich for one day. Or else "instant wealth" agencies provided papers, good only for the few hours spent in the Consulate. And, of course, despite all the pledges to return, I didn't know anyone who had any intention of coming back.

If an applicant came out of the Con-sulate smiling, the line outside collapsed as people mobbed the apparently successful candidate: "What did he ask? What did you say? What did he say?" Most people emerged with long faces and were shunned, as if they were contagious.

One morning, the visa officer turned down six consecutive doctors and told the seventh, who happened to be a friend of mine, and whom I'll call Vadivel, "Spare me the crap about coming back with specialized knowledge to serve your country. Why do you really want to go?" Vadivel, who had held on to his American dream for so long that he could speak with the passion of a visionary, said, "Sir, craving your indulgence, I want to train in a decent, ten-story hospital where the lifts are actually working. I want to pass board-certification exams by my own merit and not through pull or bribes. I want to become a wonderful doctor, practice real medicine, pay taxes, make a good living, drive a big car on decent roads, and eventually live in the Ansel Adams section of New Mexico and never come back to this wretched town, where doctors are as numerous as fleas and practice is cutthroat, and where the air outside is not even fit to breathe." The consul gave him a visa. The eighth applicant, forewarned, tried the same tactic but was turned down.

At the entrance to the internes' quarters, which occupied the top floor of a three-story building, the peon whose full-time job was to sit by the solitary phone and log the calls from the matrons and wake up the appropriate interne was snoring. A faint odor of ganja was in the air.

A door burst open and a fellow-interne, known as Mo, stumbled out of his room, almost knocking into me. He had his left hand raised above his head, and the fingers of his right were applying pressure to the antecubital vein. I guessed that Mo had mainlined with pethidine and had come out of his room so the sea breeze could fan the flames of his rush.

"Sorry, bugger," he said.

Mo was part of a different kind of madness from what we would-be foreign medical graduates went in for. He belonged to the peth-and-poker crowd. There was a room in the men's hostel where a poker game was reputed to have gone on day and night for three years—with politicians, lawyers, and other dadas coming and going, and a percentage of the kitty going to the occupant of the room. Mo, like many in his group, had been in medical school for many years, consistently failing the anatomy viva voce. He had passed and become an interne when state elections brought one of his relatives into power, giving him the necessary pull to get through.

Tonight, the pethidine had taken away the barrier that usually kept him wary of me. "Abe, you lucky bugger," he said. He lowered his arm and clamped it over my shoulder. "I wish I could go to America."

I was about to mention what many of my classmates planned to do: get a position in England or Tanzania or Nigeria or the Caribbean and from there get a visa to America, because the odds were better than in Madras. Of course, he had to study and clear the exams first.

"No, bugger," he said, anticipating my advice. "If at all I go, I'll marry a green-card holder, then live there and do Stanley Kaplan till I pass. Or maybe do business in Las Vegas or something. But, no, I think I'll stay here. Desh—mother-land—that's important to me."

His voice took on a conspiratorial tone. "I heard that one of our buggers, when he landed at Kennedy, he met a beautiful woman—a deadly blonde—and her brother outside baggage claim. She was very, very friendly. They offered him a lift in a white convertible. They took him to their apartment, and then you know what the brother did? Pulled a bloody gun out and said, 'Screw my sister or I'll kill you.' Can you imagine? What a country!"

Mo's deadly-blonde fantasy was just one version of the American dream that most of us had. And Vadivel had been right when he told the consular officer that doctors abounded in India; what was lacking was money to provide meaningful treatment to people in need. America was the land where there was no dichotomy between what the textbook said you should do and what you could do—or so we thought. In America, your talent and hard work could take you to the very top. It was the land of defibrillators on every ward and disposable everything, by God—no more mucking around in the murky waters of a lukewarm sterilizer for a needle that could actually penetrate skin. As for the deadly blonde...

I arrived in America a few months before my internship was due to start. My graduation gift from my parents had been a fifteen-day airline ticket that allowed multiple stops around America. My mood was euphoric. On my first stop, I met a friend of a friend who was just finishing his internship at an East Coast hospital. We slipped into the easy familiarity of expatriates. Over dinner at a Vietnamese restaurant, I told him the places I hoped to apply to.

He laughed. "Don't be so bloody naïve, bugger," he said. "Learn from the experience of others. Look." He pushed a chili-sauce bottle to the center of the table. "This, my dear friend, is an Ellis Island hospital. Mark my words, every city has one. Such a place is completely dependent on foreign medical graduates, and that's where you will go. No ifs and buts. Think of it as a quarantine period, before you can move on and do your land-of-opportunity fantasy. Your elders and betters have passed through these places. Why should you think you are different?"

Now he put a saltshaker as far away from the chili-sauce bottle as he could. "That," he said, "is a Plymouth Rock hospital—university- and medical-school-affiliated, of course. It has never taken a foreign medical graduate. Except for the occasional South African white or Brit or Australian, who—don't ask why—is a different species of foreign medical graduate from you and me. Don't even bother with that kind of place. The cowpath from India never goes through there. Unless you want to take a job as a bathroom sweeper."

He could see that I resisted this argument, and my resistance irritated him. "Look here. We foreign medical graduates are an embarrassment to this society, a problem," he said, waggling the index and middle fingers of both hands, as if placing quotation marks—a gesture I'd never seen in India. "We are like the Mexican-migrant-worker problem, or the Colombian-cocaine-export problem. Alas, we problems wouldn't exist if the United States economy didn't depend on us, if there wasn't a great need for the commodity we provide and which they are willing to pay for. They create the problem. But that doesn't mean they have to like us, or treat us fairly."

He signalled for the check. "We are, my dear friend, like a transplanted organ—lifesaving, and desperately needed, but rejected because we are foreign tissue. But, as they say in America, tough shit."

Contrariness made me visit a Plymouth Rock hospital in Boston. The secretary in the internal-medicine office was barely cordial. She soon ascertained what my appearance had already suggested: that I was a foreign medical graduate. I explained that, since I had never received a reply to my letter of inquiry, I thought that perhaps their letter to me had been lost in the mail. "Not likely," she said. There was a long silence.

A wiser traveller, I continued my journey across America. I discovered that the patient population at a Plymouth Rock hospital was not necessarily different from that at an Ellis Island hospital. What ultimately stigmatized an Ellis Island hospital was not its patients but its doctors. The very fact that it had become dependent on foreign medical graduates made American medical students avoid the place. At Ellis Island hospitals, I was welcomed by the secretaries in the residency offices and had interviews with program directors who were eager to sign me up. I thought that I could read their thoughts: Hmm...speaks well...not much of an accent...more of a British accent, if anything, great exam scores...not the never-raise-the-toilet-seat, spit-out-of- the-window type.

I applied to a new medical school—East Tennessee State University, in Johnson City, Tennessee, in the foothill of the Smoky Mountains. The residency program was so new that it had not clearly defined itself as foreign-medical-graduate-dependent or not. I was given a contract. My fellow-internes included a couple of Americans as well as foreign medical graduates from India, the Philippines, and Haiti.

On the first day of orientation, I was nervous. But nothing about the wards, the lab, the medical library, or the intensive-care unit was unexpected. I had simply arrived in the very situation I had visualized for years. I loved the way the charts were kept, with tabs separating order sheets, progress notes, laboratory results, nurses' notes, radiological reports, and consultants' notes. A call to the medical-record department would bring two or three volumes of the patient's old chart. By studying these, one could reconstruct the waxing and waning of a disease over time. And after I discharged the patient I could follow him regularly in the outpatient clinic and add to the chronicle of his encounter with illness. I had been right about one thing in America: what you should do for a patient, you could do.

I was intensely aware of myself at all times. I realized that I was trying not to stand out, and would speak in a manner that was understood, even if it meant pronouncing gastroenterology in one slurred ejaculation, rather than "gastroenterology." I asked my senior resident, John Duncan, to show me how to tie my necktie in a thinner knot than the broad seventies knot I used. I studied sociological minutiae carefully, even keeping notes in my diary on the etiquette of the cafeteria line—how queue-jumping was permissible if you were heading for the salad bar, how having money ready when you got to the cashier was appreciated, how the sawdust-tasting entity appropriately called grits was to be avoided, how biscuits and gravy were tasty but sat in your belly like bricks, and, most important, where the Tabasco sauce was kept. Tabasco provided the only way I could keep my taste buds from atrophying completely. I wanted my foreignness to be forgotten. The highest compliment I received after three months of this was paid me by a nurse: she said, "Doc, I don't know where you're from, but you're a good ole Tennessee boy in my book. Are you married?"

Each year in Tennessee, I encountered more second-generation Indians in the medical-school classes. I was fascinated by the contrast between their looks and their manner. It was like a trick of some sort—how, when they opened their mouths, the most fluent East Tennessee patois emerged. I thought (and perhaps I was wrong) that they were so American, so assimilated, that they had a confidence, a swagger, that we first-generation immigrants would never have. The F.M.G.s jokingly, and jealously, referred to them as A.B.C.D.s: American-Born Confused Deshis.

In the third year of my medical residency, I spent my free weekends working in small emergency rooms in tiny towns tucked away in the Appalachian Mountains. The staff physicians in these little mining communities were mostly Indians, with a smattering of other foreign medical graduates. The few American doctors there were usually hometown boys who had returned after their training. I studied the Indian doctors: they represented a later stage in the life cycle of a foreign medical graduate.

One of these doctors invited me to his house. His wife and children were on vacation in India. We had a couple of beers. He seemed lonely, sinking deeper into his recliner as the evening wore on, his every sentence tinged with nostalgia. It struck me that in the privacy of his home he was more Indian than he might have been in India. If I was trying to integrate, and learn the rituals of Monday-night football and Moon Pies, cookouts and coon-hunting, squirrel stew and pos-sum pie, this doctor had abandoned that strategy. Or else he had worked his way through that phase and arrived at this.

On the walls of his den were pictures of his family. "That's my oldest daughter, he said, pointing. "Guess what—-she's been accepted by Harvard as an undergraduate. Pre-med, of course."

His face revealed more than just parental pride. He wanted her to succeed in a way that he, for all his financial success, never could. His daughter would soon penetrate the upper tier of medicine, which had been closed to him. She would step right into it, as if it were her birthright—sans accent and with an American medical degree. There was pride and vindication in his expression.

I wasn't ready to settle in the hinterland. I wanted to make it to Plymouth Rock. My mentor in Tennessee, an infectious-disease specialist named Steven Berk, had sparked my interest in that field and encouraged me to apply for a fellowship. Once again, in 1982, I sent out applications to the best programs in the country. But this time I actually received replies.

I asked myself what had changed. I had published a few papers by then, but Berk's strong letter of recommendation had helped; it said, "Look beyond the foreign-medical-graduate label." When Boston University made me a preëmptive offer of a fellowship, before the official "match" day, I accepted. I had finally penetrated the country club.

Boston was Mecca. It had three medical schools, each with years of tradition, and each owning or linked to several famous hospitals. I sat in lecture halls listening to speakers whose papers and textbook chapters I had read and who had been mythical figures to me. My fellow-trainees—all American graduates—found my propensity for hero worship amusing. Real fame in Boston that year belonged to Ray Flynn, Yo-Yo Ma, and Larry Bird.

Half of my fellowship training was spent in laboratory research, learning basic techniques. I embarked on a study of pneumonia using an animal model. The laboratory skills and the imagination required to be a first-class researcher were quite distinct from the skills demanded of a clinician. Either you had them or you didn't.

I soon noticed that in Boston, as in Tennessee, there wasn't much interest in the bedside exam. Most case discussions took place in conference rooms or labs. As a student in India, I had imagined that the ready availability of CAT scans and angiograms, the routine ability to float Swan-Ganz catheters into the heart and measure pressures, and so on, would have resulted in American doctors' becoming

superb bedside sleuths. They had so many opportunities to confirm bedside findings with appropriate investigations. But instead their senses were rusty from lack
of use, and there was little faith in the bedside exam.

I realized that the movers and shakers in medicine—the chairmen and the department heads with the magnificent titles—didn't get to their positions by seeing
patients. Their fame and power had come from doing basic biological research, at
which they were brilliant. American education, unlike didactic Indian education,
encouraged innovative and original thinking, and this was where it paid off: if
medicine was both art and science, no country in the world was better at the science than America. Typically, early in these doctors' careers they had explored and
described an important phenomenon and written the seminal paper on it. They
had then spent years refining that observation and assigning Younger Turks to
pursue the spinoffs, all the while broadening their sphere of influence, writing
textbook chapters on the subject, sitting on the National Institutes of Health and
Veterans Administration committees that awarded funding. The necessary skills
for such a rise were business acumen, Machiavellian cunning, and skill in the
thrust-and-parry action of committees. And all the while the research ship had to
be kept afloat. If you were looking for an outstanding clinician, someone whom
other doctors would seek if they were ill, it was unlikely that you would find one
in a position of power.

One of the professors I admired the most was a superb clinician and a gifted
researcher. He let me run the clinical service without much interference. I presented the new consultations to him every afternoon, in his lab. Almost never did I
present a patient with a condition that he hadn't seen before. On one occasion, I
surprised him by something I'd said.

"That's just not possible, Abe," he said. "It can't be." He wanted to see the patient.
Our entourage marched over to the hospital. The professor, wrapped up in his
thoughts, extended his hand. The patient, thinking that this meant a hand-shake,
extended hers. But the professor's fingers had already slipped past the outstretched hand to grab the bedsheet and expose the part of the body in question,
to see for himself what it was that seemed to defy his knowledge of how this particular disease worked. He showed us what we had missed—a finding that we
thought was trivial but that was, in fact, crucial. He marched out, satisfied, having
proved what it was that he had come to prove: that the rules of how infections
behaved had not been broken. He left us to explain to the astonished patient that
she had just received the opinion of the top infectious-disease expert in America.

I began to understand that if I still aspired to one of the heady titles that I had fantasized about as a student my life would have to take a path I hadn't anticipated. After two years, my research had barely begun to yield results. It would take several more years of committed laboratory apprenticeship before I could start exploring the research questions that really interested me. I had gone into medicine partly because middle-class Indian parents guided their children into either engineering or medicine, as if there were no other careers. But I had also chosen medicine because of Somerset Maugham's "Of Human Bondage," a book that when I was thirteen made medicine seem the most romantic of professions: "humanity there in the rough, the materials the artist worked on," in Maugham's words. In medical school Professor K.V.T. had embodied this approach to medicine for me. I was reluctant now to change paths. I had started to resent the time I was spending away from my patients. A new disease, AIDS, had emerged. While re-searchers chased after its cause, there was plenty of opportunity for a clinician to observe its manifestations at the bedside. I wanted to combine patient care and teaching with more modest research.

I had made the passage from India to Plymouth Rock. But there I discovered that one of the most important things America had to offer was the choice of how one could live and work.

After finishing my fellowship, in 1985, I went back to India. It was a nostalgic visit to see friends and relatives; my return ticket was safely in my pocket. Nevertheless, I wanted to find out whether India would feel different. I had a fleeting fantasy that I might discover a way of using my specialty in infectious diseases within India.

I carried with me an old but functioning gastroscope donated by a physician in Tennessee; I was to deliver it to a Methodist mission hospital in the state of Karnataka which was supported by an American congregation. But the customs officers in Bombay wouldn't release the gastroscope; they were convinced that I wanted to sell it. At the time, India had huge taxes on most imported items. I argued to no avail. The gastroscope never left customs and is probably still sitting there. I visited the isolated rural mission hospital anyway. The senior doctor, an ophthalmologist; had given his best years to the hospital. He was dedicated but poorly paid. His strong religious belief—something I lacked—was what kept him there. In the same hospital, I met a young anesthetist and his obstetrician wife, both fresh out of training. I thought that they were wonderful, compassionate physicians. But as their child neared school age they worried about the lack of good schools in the village. Their pay was insufficient to buy even the simplest luxuries that India's huge middle class took for granted. I couldn't see them stay-ing there for more than another year or so. I couldn't see myself working there, either.

On a subsequent visit, four years later, I noted a new phenomenon sweeping Madras and other cities in India: N.R.I. hospitals. These were nonresident-Indian hospitals, set up by Indian doctors living abroad who invested their foreign exchange in hospitals modeled on their counterparts in the West, right down to the modular furniture in the foyers. These hospitals offered everything from renal transplants to coronary-bypass surgery. But they were expensive and catered to the rich. The very rich, however, still went to Manhattan's Sloan-Kettering or the Texas Heart Institute.

I made rounds at one of these hospitals for two weeks. I gave a formal lecture. And I tried to imagine myself living and working in this setting, but I couldn't. I made excuses for myself on the plane returning to America. "No one knows what to do with your specialty in India," I told myself. "Most physicians manage the infections they encounter without outside assistance, and they're not about to change to help you make a living. And, as for AIDS, Abe, they seem to think that it is and will remain an American problem. Money is the missing ingredient in India, not you. You're just not needed, Abe. If a new enlightened government ever comes along ..." I never completely convinced myself.

My academic career, spent largely in smaller medical schools where patient care was valued more than research, brought me, eventually, to America's southern-most border—to a professorship at the Texas Tech University Health Sciences Center, in El Paso, and to a consultancy at R. E. Thomason Hospital, a county hos-pital. For the first time in America, I felt as if I had disappeared. I no longer stood out. The patients and their families walking the corridors of the county hospital looked like my kin from South India. They shared my skin color and took me to be Hispanic. When I was stopped in the corridors and asked questions in Spanish, I learned to respond with answers such as "La cafeteria es en el basement"—bor-der Spanglish, allowing one the liberty of throwing in English when nothing else could do the job. A sizable percentage of our patients were Mexican nationals. The hospital required only an El Paso billing address to provide service. As the sole not-for-profit hospital serving a population of almost seven hundred thousand, well over a third of whom were uninsured, we were overburdened and under-staffed. But you'd have known this only if you read it somewhere. The wards were airy, and sunlight from big picture windows flooded the corridors, reflecting off the waxed floors and pale-blue walls of the internal-medicine ward. The security guards directed you to the choice ca/do de res and barbacoa joints on Alameda Avenue; the nurses smiled, and if they felt embattled they didn't show it. As a doctor interested in infectious diseases, I had found a perfect niche in El Paso: treating Third World diseases —typhoid, amoebic liver abscesses, brucellosis—in a First World setting.

In 1993, I found myself in the South of India again, this time at the Oberoi Hotel in Bangalore, and I was having a strange conversation with the bellman. The annual struggle to fill our internship slots at Texas Tech had become desperate. Despite the fact that our medical students loved the experience at the county hospital, they had no intention of staying with us as internes. We had always been dependent on foreign medical graduates, and it appeared that we always would be. But visas for foreign medical graduates, which seemed to have been easier to obtain at the peak of the AIDS epidemic, were once again difficult to get. A new twist had been added: to have a chance for a visa, you had to have a contract with a residency program in America.

I had come to India to interview potential internes, pick the best, and hand out five contracts. These five graduates, contract in hand, would have a decent chance of getting their visas. Before I left El Paso, I had run a small ad in an Indian newspaper, specifying a very high score on the equivalency exam. I thought that I would get ten or twenty applicants. Four hundred people answered the advertisement, all of them meeting or exceeding the qualifications and overwhelming the fax machine in El Paso. I had picked seventy people to interview in Bangalore.

The bellman at the Oberoi was a bright young man, and it didn't surprise me when he told me he had a college degree. He hoped to rise in the catering field, he said. It had good prospects overseas.

"There have been many people inquiring about you, sir. Starting three days ago," the bellman said.

"What do they want to know?"

"How you look. Whether you seem strict or not." He grinned.

"What else?"

"Just silly people…"

"Tell me."

"One fellow asked…I'm ashamed to tell you."

"Go ahead."

"He asked whether you are susceptible to …"

"To what?"

" 'Monetary adjustments'—his exact words, sir, I swear."

"Well, I'm not. Spread the word."

"If you don't mind my suggesting, sir, leave a list with our telephone operator of people whose calls you want put through. She will not connect other calls." I must have looked puzzled, because he went on to say, "Otherwise, ministers and what-not will be bothering you all night."

The lobby of the hotel the next morning looked like a variant of the Consulate scene. Even though I had given each person a specific time to appear over the next two days, it looked as if they were all there.

The hotel made its business suite available to me, and I began to work my way through the applicants. The secretary assisting me told me that people I had finished interviewing were being mobbed outside. "What did he ask? What did you say?" My questions were designed simply to get to know the candidates and to pick out the brightest, smartest ones. But now, as an experiment, I began deliberately throwing in specific questions, such as "How do you feel about Clinton?" and "What are your views on homosexuality?" By the afternoon, I was getting polished but totally noncommittal answers to these questions, since nobody had any idea what my views were.

I asked one young man why he wanted to leave.

"I want to specialize in hematology oncology and then return to serve—"

"Save that for the Consulate. Really, why do you want to leave?"

He was startled. After a moment's silence, his face broke out into a naughty smile.

"You know, sir," he said. I did, but I wanted to hear anyway. Reluctantly, almost ashamed, he went on, "It's just hopeless—that's all I can tell you, sir. No jobs. And to get into specialty training here requires influence. And there are so many medical schools now that having a specialty degree here means less and less. And if you join government service, without some political pull you will be posted to some godforsaken place forever. And to set up a private practice—it's cutthroat, sir. Unless you have a rich father-in-law who builds a hospital for you."

According to him, yet another wrinkle had been added to the protocol of leaving: you had to have an N.O.C.—a no-objection certificate—which showed that India didn't mind your decamping. This seemed to me to be a brilliant obstacle set up by the Indian government to plug the brain drain. "But," he reassured me quickly, "N.O.C.s are no problem. They are easily obtained by lubricating the right person in Delhi."

I asked him why it was that all those I had interviewed so far claimed to want to pursue hematology-oncology after their residency in internal medicine.

"It's because that's the only category of subspecialty training not readily available in India, sir. Therefore, technically, an N.O.C. can be issued. That's why we say that to you, sir." He had dropped all pretense now. He was giving me the inside story. "Everyone tells the consular officer that he wants to return and start a bone-marrow-transplant center in India. The consular officer said to someone the other day that if everyone who said that actually came back India would have more bone-marrow-transplant centers than chai shops."

By the evening of the second day, I had my five candidates. I was exhausted. The gruelling process of talking to so many young doctors, and hearing why they wanted to leave, had given me a sense of being immensely fortunate—fortunate that my parents had emigrated, fortunate that I had got the residency in Tennessee, fortunate in my choice of specialty.

My journey to America had brought me full circle, back to India, and to a situation where I could pick others to make the voyage. The best I could do for the five doctors I had picked was to bring them to a county hospital like mine: Ellis Island. The rest was up to them.

On Not Winning the Nobel Prize

Doris Lessing

I am standing in a doorway looking through clouds of blowing dust to where I am told there is still uncut forest. Yesterday I drove through miles of stumps, and charred remains of fires where in '56 was the most wonderful forest I have ever seen, all destroyed. People have to eat. They have to get fuel for fires.

This is north west Zimbabwe early in the eighties, and I am visiting a friend who was a teacher in a school in London. He is here "to help Africa" as we put it. He is a gently idealistic soul and what he found here in this school shocked him into a depression, from which it was hard to recover. This school is like all the schools built after Independence. It consists of four large brick rooms side by side, put straight into the dust, one two three four, with a half room at one end, which is the library. In these classrooms are blackboards, but my friend keeps the chalks in his pocket, as otherwise they would be stolen. There is no atlas, or globe in the school, no textbooks, no exercise books, or biros, in the library are no books of the kind the pupils would like to read: they are tomes from American universities, hard even to lift, rejects from white libraries, detective stories, or with titles like 'Weekend in Paris' or 'Felicity Finds Love'.

There is a goat trying to find sustenance in some aged grass. The headmaster has embezzled the school funds and is suspended, arousing the question familiar to all of us but usually in more august contexts: How is it these people behave like this when they must know everyone is watching them?

My friend doesn't have any money because everyone, pupils and teachers, borrow from him when he is paid and will probably never pay it back. The pupils range from six to twenty-six, because some who did not get schooling earlier are here to make it up. Some pupils walk every morning many miles, rain or shine and across rivers. They cannot do homework because there is no electricity in the villages, and you can't study easily by the light of a burning log. The girls have to fetch water and cook when they get home from school and before they set off for school.

As I sit with my friend in his room, people drop shyly in, and all, everyone begs for books. "Please send us books when you get back to London". One man said, "They taught us to read but we have no books". Everybody I met, everyone, begged for books.

I was there some days. The dust blew past, water was short because the pumps had broken and the women were getting water from the river again.

Another idealistic teacher from England was rather ill after seeing what this "school" was like.

On the last day, it was end of term and they slaughtered the goat, and it was cut into mounds of bits and cooked in a great tin. This was the much looked forward to end of term feast, boiled goat and porridge. I drove away while it was going on, back through the charred remains and stumps of the forest.

I do not think many of the pupils of this school will get prizes.

Next day I am at a school in North London, a very good school, whose name we all know. It is a school for boys. Good buildings, and gardens.

These pupils have a visit from some well known person every week, and it is in the nature of things that these may be fathers, relatives, even mothers of the pupils. A visit from a celebrity is no big deal for them.

The school in the blowing dust of northwest Zimbabwe is in my mind, and I look at those mildly expectant faces and try to tell them about what I have seen in the last week. Classrooms without books, without text books, or an atlas, or even a map pinned up on a wall. A school where the teachers beg to be sent books to tell them how to teach, they being only eighteen or nineteen themselves, they beg for books. I tell these boys that everybody, everyone begs for books: "Please send us books". I am sure that everyone here, making a speech will know that moment when the faces you are looking at are blank. Your listeners cannot hear what you are saying: there are no images in their minds to match what you are telling them. In this case, of a school standing in dust clouds, where water is short, and where, at the end of term, a just killed goat cooked in a great pot is the end of term treat.

Is it really so impossible for them to imagine such bare poverty?

I do my best. They are polite.

I'm pretty sure of this lot there will be some who will win prizes.

Then, it is over, and I with the teachers, ask as always, how the library is, and if the pupils read. And here, in this privileged school, I hear what I always hear when I go to schools and even universities.

"You know how it is. A lot of the boys have never read at all, and the library is only half used."

"You know how it is." Yes, we indeed do know how it is. All of us.

We are in a fragmenting culture, where our certainties of even a few decades ago are questioned and where it is common for young men and women who have had years of education, to know nothing about the world, to have read nothing, knowing only some speciality or other, for instance, computers.

What has happened to us is an amazing invention, computers and the internet and TV, a revolution. This is not the first revolution we, the human race, has dealt with. The printing revolution, which did not take place in a matter of a few decades, but took much longer, changed our minds and ways of thinking. A foolhardy lot, we accepted it all, as we always do, never asked "What is going to happen to us now, with this invention of print?" And just as we never once stopped to ask, How are we, our minds, going to change with the new internet, which has seduced a whole generation into its inanities so that even quite reasonable people will confess that once they are hooked, it is hard to cut free, and they may find a whole day has passed in blogging and blugging etc.

Very recently, anyone even mildly educated would respect learning, education, and owe respect to our great store of literature. Of course we all know that when this happy state was with us, people would pretend to read, would pretend respect for learning, but it is on record that working men and women longed for books, and this is evidenced by the working men's libraries, institutes, colleges of the 18th and 19th centuries.

Reading, books, used to be part of a general education.

Older people, talking to young ones, must understand just how much of an education it was, reading, because the young ones know so much less. And if children cannot read, it is because they have not read.

But we all know this sad story.

But we do not know the end of it.

We think of the old adage, "Reading maketh a full man" – and forgetting about jokes to do with over-eating – reading makes a woman and a man full of information, of history, of all kinds of knowledge.

But we are not the only people in the world. Not long ago I was telephoned by a friend who said she had been in Zimbabwe, in a village where they had not eaten for three days, but they were talking about books and how to get them, about education.

I belong to a little organisation which started out with the intention of getting books into the villages. There was a group of people who in another connection had travelled Zimbabwe at its grass roots. They reported that the villages, unlike what people reported, are full of intelligent people, teachers retired, teachers on leave, children on holidays, old people. I myself paid for a little survey, of what people wanted to read, and found the results were the same as a Swedish survey, that I had not known about. People wanted to read what people in Europe want to read, if they read at all – novels of all kinds, science fiction, poetry, detective fiction, plays, Shakespeare, and the do-it-yourself books, like how to open a bank account, were low in the list. All of Shakespeare: they knew the name. A problem with finding books for villagers is that they don't know what is available, so a school set book, like the Mayor of Casterbridge, becomes popular because they know it is there. Animal Farm, for obvious reasons is the most popular of all novels.

Our little organisation got books from where we could, but remember that a good paperback from England cost a months wages: that was before Mugabe's reign of terror. Now with inflation, it would cost several years wages. But having taken a box of books out to a village – and remember there is a terrible shortage of petrol, the box will be greeted with tears. The library may be a plank under a tree on bricks. And within a week there will be literacy classes – people who can read teaching those who can't, citizenship class – and in one remote village, since there were no novels in Tonga, a couple of lads sat down to write novels in Tonga. There are six or so main languages in Zimbabwe and there are novels in all of them, violent, incestuous, full of crime and murder.

Our little organisation was supported from the very start by Norway, and then by Sweden. But without this kind of support our supplies of books would have dried up. Novels published in Zimbabwe, and, too, do-it-yourself books are sent out to people who thirst for them.

It is said that a people gets the government it deserves, but I do not think it is true of Zimbabwe. And we must remember that this respect and hunger for books comes, not from Mugabe's regime, but from the one before it, the whites. It is an astonishing phenomenon, this hunger for books, and it can be seen everywhere from Kenya down to the Cape of Good Hope.

This links up improbably with a fact: I was brought up in what was virtually a mud hut, thatched. This house has been built always, everywhere, where there are reeds or grass, suitable mud, poles for walls. Saxon England for example. The one I was brought up in had four rooms, one beside another, not one, and, the point is, it was full of books. Not only did my parents take books from England to Africa, but my mother ordered books from England for her children, books in great brown paper parcels which were the joy of my young life. A mud hut, but full of books.

And sometimes I get letters from people living in a village that might not have electricity or running water (just like our family in our elongated mud hut), "I shall be a writer too, because I've the same kind of house you were in."

But here is the difficulty. No.

Writing, writers, do not come out of houses without books.

There is the gap. There is the difficulty.

I have been looking at the speeches by some of your recent prizewinners. Take the magnificent Pamuk. He said his father had 1 500 books. His talent did not come out of the air, he was connected with the great tradition.

Take V.S. Naipaul. He mentions that the Indian Vedas were close behind the memory of his family. His father encouraged him to write. And when he got to England by right he used the British Library. So he was close to the great tradition.

Let us take John Coetzee. He was not only close to the great tradition, he was the tradition: he taught literature in Cape Town. And how sorry I am that I was never in one of his classes: taught by that wonderfully brave bold mind.

In order to write, in order to make literature, there must be a close connection with libraries, books, the Tradition.

I have a friend from Zimbabwe. A writer. Black – and that is to the point. He taught himself to read from the labels on jam jars, the labels on preserved fruit cans. He was brought up in an area I have driven through, an area for rural blacks. The earth is grit and gravel, there are low sparse bushes. The huts are poor, nothing like the good cared-for huts of the better off. A school – but like one I have described. He found a discarded children's encyclopaedia on a rubbish heap and learned from it.

On Independence in 1980 there was a group of good writers in Zimbabwe, truly a nest of singing birds. They were bred in old Southern Rhodesia, under the whites – the mission schools, the better schools. Writers are not made in Zimbabwe. Not easily, not under Mugabe.

All the writers had a difficult road to literacy, let alone being writers. I would say print on jam tins and discarded encyclopaedias were not uncommon. And we are talking about people hungering for standards of education they were a long way from. A hut or huts with many children – an overworked mother, a fight for food and clothing.

Yet despite these difficulties, writers came into being, and there is another thing we should remember. This was Zimbabwe, physically conquered less than a hundred years before. The grandfathers and grandmothers of these people might have been storytellers for their clan. The oral tradition. In one generation – two, the transition from stories remembered and passed on, to print, to books. What an achievement.

Books, literally wrested from rubbish heaps and the detritus of the white man's world. But you may have a sheaf of paper (not typescript – that is a book – but it has to find a publisher, who will then pay you, remain solvent, distribute the books. I have had several accounts sent to me of the publishing scene for Africa. Even in more privileged places like North Africa, with its different tradition, to talk of a publishing scene is a dream of possibilities.

Here I am talking about books never written, writers that could not make it because the publishers are not there. Voices unheard. It is not possible to estimate this great waste of talent, of potential. But even before that stage of a book's creation which demands a publisher, an advance, encouragement, there is something else lacking.

Writers are often asked, How do you write? With a processor? an electric typewriter? a quill? longhand? But the essential question is, "Have you found a space, that empty space, which should surround you when you write? Into that space, which is like a form of listening, of attention, will come the words, the words your characters will speak, ideas – inspiration.

If this writer cannot find this space, then poems and stories may be stillborn.

When writers talk to each other, what they ask each other is always to do with this space, this other time. "Have you found it? Are you holding it fast?"

Let us jump to an apparently very different scene. We are in London, one of the big cities. There is a new writer. We, cynically enquire, How are her boobs? Is she good-looking? If this is a man, Charismatic? Handsome? We joke but it is not a joke.

This new find is acclaimed, possibly given a lot of money. The buzzing of paparazzi begins in their poor ears. They are feted, lauded, whisked about the world. Us old ones, who have seen it all, are sorry for this neophyte, who has no idea of what is really happening.

He, she is flattered, pleased.

But ask in a year's time what he or she is thinking: I've heard them: "This is the worst thing that could have happened to me."

Some much publicised new writers haven't written again, or haven't written what they wanted to, meant to.

And we, the old ones, want to whisper into those innocent ears. "Have you still got your space? Your sole, your own and necessary place where your own voices may speak to you, you alone, where you may dream. Oh, hold onto it, don't let it go."

There must be some kind of education.

My mind is full of splendid memories of Africa which I can revive and look at when I want. How about those sunsets, gold and purple and orange, spreading across the sky at evening. How about butterflies and moths and bees on the aromatic bushes of the Kalahari? Or, sitting on the banks of the Zambesi, where it rolls between pale grassy banks, it being the dry season, dark-green and glossy, with all the birds of Africa around its banks. Yes, elephants, giraffes, lions and the rest, there were plenty of those, but how about the sky at night, still unpolluted, black and wonderful, full of restless stars.

But there are other memories. A young man, eighteen perhaps, is in tears, standing in his "library." A visiting American seeing a library without books, sent a crate, but this young man took each one out, reverently, and wrapped them in plastic. "But," we say, "these books were sent to be read, surely?" and he replied, "No, they will get dirty, and where will I get anymore?"

He wants us to send him books from England to teach him to teach. "I only did four years in the senior school" he begs, "But they never taught me to teach."

I have seen a Teacher in a school where there was no textbooks, not even a bit of chalk for the blackboard – it was stolen – teach his class of six to eighteen year olds by moving stones in the dust, chanting "Two times two is....." and so on. I have seen a girl, perhaps not more than twenty, similarly lacking textbooks, exercise books, biros – anything, teach the A, B, C in the dust with a stick, while the sun beat down and the dust swirled.

We are seeing here that great hunger for education in Africa, anywhere in the Third World, or whatever we call parts of the world where parents long to get an education for their children which will take them from poverty, to the advantage of an education.

Our education which is so threatened now.

I would like you to imagine yourselves, somewhere in Southern Africa, standing in an Indian store, in a poor area, in a time of bad drought. There is a line of people, mostly women, with every kind of container for water. This store gets a bowser of water every afternoon from the town and the people are waiting for this precious water.

The Indian is standing with the heels of his hands pressed down on the counter, and he is watching a black woman, who is bending over a wadge of paper that looks as if it has been torn out of a book. She is reading Anna Karenin.

She is reading slowly, mouthing the words. It looks a difficult book. This is a young woman with two little children clutching at her legs. She is pregnant. The Indian is distressed, because the young woman's headscarf, which should be white, is yellow with dust. Dust lies between her breasts and on her arms. This man is distressed because of the lines of people, all thirsty, but he doesn't have enough water for them. He is angry because he knows there are people dying out there, beyond the dust clouds. His brother, older, had been here holding the fort, but he had said he needed a break, had gone into town, really rather ill, because of the drought.

This man is curious. He says to the young woman. "What are you reading?"

"It is about Russia," says the girl.

"Do you know where Russia is?" He hardly knows himself.

The young woman looks straight at him, full of dignity though her eyes are red from dust, "I was best in the class. My teacher said, I was best."

The young woman resumes her reading: she wants to get to the end of the paragraph.

The Indian looks at the two little children and reaches for some Fanta, but the mother says "Fanta makes them thirsty."

The Indian knows he shouldn't do this but he reaches down to a great plastic container beside him, behind the counter and pours out two plastic mugs of water, which he hands to the children. He watches while the girl looks at her children drinking, her mouth moving. He gives her a mug of water. It hurts him to see her drinking it, so painfully thirsty is she.

Now she hands over to him a plastic water container, which he fills. The young woman and the children, watch him closely so that he doesn't spill any.

She is bending again over the book. She reads slowly but the paragraph fascinates her and she reads it again.

"Varenka, with her white kerchief over her black hair, surrounded by the children and gaily and good-humouredly busy with them, and at the same visibly excited at the possibility of an offer of marriage from a man she cared for, looked very attractive. Koznyshev walked by her side and kept casting admiring glances at her. Looking at her, he recalled all the delightful things he had heard from her lips, all the good he knew about her, and became more and more conscious that the feeling he had for her was something rare, something he had felt but once before, long, long ago, in his early youth. The joy of being near her increased step by step, and at last reached such a point that, as he put a huge birch mushroom with a slender stalk and up-curling top into her basket, he looked into her eyes and, noting the flush of glad and frightened agitation that suffused her face, he was confused himself, and in silence gave her a smile that said too much."

This lump of print is lying on the counter, together with some old copies of magazines, some pages of newspapers, girls in bikinis.

It is time for her to leave the haven of the Indian store, and set off back along the four miles to her village. It is time... outside the lines of waiting women clamour and complain. But still the Indian lingers. He knows what it will cost this girl – going back home, with the two clinging children. He would give her the piece of prose that so fascinates her, but he cannot really believe this splinter of a girl with her great belly can really understand it.

Why is perhaps a third of Anna Karenin stuck here on this counter in a remote Indian store? It is like this.

A certain high official, United Nations, as it happens, bought a copy of this novel in the bookshop when he set out on his journeys to cross several oceans and seas. On the plane, settled in his business class seat, he tore the book into three parts. He looks around at his fellow passengers as he does this, knowing he will see looks of shock, curiosity, but some of amusement. When he was settled, his seat belt tight, he said aloud to whoever could hear, "I always do this when I've a long trip. You don't want to have to hold up some heavy great book." The novel was a paperback, but, true, it is a long book. This man is well used to people listening when he spoke. "I always do this, travelling," he confided. "Travelling at all these days, is hard enough." And as soon as people were settling down, he opened his part of Anna Karenin, and read. When people looked his way, curiously or not, he confided in them. "No, it is really the only way to travel." He knew the novel, liked it, and this original mode of reading did add spice to what was after all a well known book.

When he reached the end of a section of the book, he called the airhostess, and sent it back to his secretary, travelling in the cheaper seats. This caused much interest, condemnation, certainly curiosity, every time a section of the great Russian novel arrived, mutilated, but readable, in the back part of the plane. Altogether, this clever way of reading Anna Karenin makes an impression, and probably no one there would forget it.

Meanwhile down in the Indian store, the young woman is holding onto the counter, her little children clinging to her skirts. She wears jeans, since she is a modern woman, but over them she had put on the heavy woollen skirt, part of traditional garb of her people: her children can easily cling onto it, the thick folds.

She sent a thankful look at the Indian, whom she knew liked her and was sorry for her, and she stepped out into the blowing clouds.

The children had gone past crying, and their throats were full of dust anyway.

This was hard, oh yes, it was hard, this stepping, one foot after another, through the dust that lay in soft deceiving mounds under her feet. Hard, hard – but she was used to hardship, was she not? Her mind was on the story she had been reading. She was thinking, "She is just like me, in her white headscarf, and she is looking after children, too. I could be her, that Russian girl. And the man there, he loves her and will ask her to marry him. (She had not finished more than that one paragraph) Yes, and a man will come for me, and take me away from all this, take me and the children, yes, he will love me and look after me."

She steps on. The can of water is heavy on her shoulders. On she goes. The children can hear the water slop in the can. Half way she stops, sets down the can. Her children are whimpering and touching the can. She thinks that she cannot open it, because dust would blow in. There is no way she can open the can until she gets home.

"Wait" she tells her children, "Wait"

She has to pull herself together and go on.

She thinks. My teacher said there was a library there, bigger than the supermarket, a big building and it is full of books. The young woman is smiling as she moves on, the dust blowing in her face. I am clever, she thinks. Teacher said I am clever. The cleverest in the school – she said I was. My children will be clever, like me. I will take them to the library, the place full of books, and they will go to school, and they will be teachers – my teacher told me I could be a teacher. They will be far from here, earning money. They will live near the big library and live a good life.

You may ask how that piece of the Russian novel ever ended up on that counter in the Indian store?

It would make a pretty story. Perhaps someone will tell it.

On goes that poor girl, held upright by thoughts of the water she would give her children once home, and drink a little herself. On she goes ... through the dreaded dusts of an African drought.

We are a jaded lot, we in our world – our threatened world. We are good for irony and even cynicism. Some words and ideas we hardly use, so worn out have they become. But we may want to restore some words that have lost their potency.

We have a treasure-house – a treasure – of literature, going back to the Egyptians, the Greeks, the Romans. It is all there, this wealth of literature, to be discovered again and again by whoever is lucky enough to come on it. A treasure. Suppose it did not exist. How impoverished, how empty we would be.

We own a legacy of languages, poems, histories, and it is not one that will ever be exhausted. It is there, always.

We have a bequest of stories, tales from the old storytellers, some of whose names we know, but some not. The storytellers go back and back, to a clearing in the forest where a great fire burns, and the old shamans dance and sing, for our heritage of stories began in fire, magic, the spirit world. And that is where it is held, today.

Ask any modern storyteller, and they will say there is always a moment when they are touched with fire, with what we like to call inspiration and this goes back and back to the beginning of our race, fire, ice and the great winds that shaped us and our world.

The storyteller is deep inside everyone of us. The story-maker is always with us. Let us suppose our world is attacked by war, by the horrors that we all of us easily imagine. Let us suppose floods wash through our cities, the seas rise ... but the sto-

ryteller will be there, for it is our imaginations which shape us, keep us, create us –
for good and for ill. It is our stories, the storyteller, that will recreate us, when we
are torn, hurt, even destroyed. It is the storyteller, the dream-maker, the myth-
maker, that is our phoenix, what we are at our best, when we are our most creative.

That poor girl trudging through the dust, dreaming of an education for her
children, do we think that we are better than she is – we, stuffed full of food, our
cupboards full of clothes, stifling in our superfluities?

I think it is that girl and the women who were talking about books and an education when they had not eaten for three days, that may yet define us.

from White Castle

Orhan Pamuk

Plague had broken in the city! Since he said this as if speaking of some other, far away place, not of Istanbul, I didn't believe it at first; I asked how he'd heard the news, I wanted to know everything. The number of sudden deaths was rising for no apparent reason, presumably caused by some disease. I asked what the signs of illness were – perhaps it wasn't plague after all. Hoja laughed at me: I shouldn't worry, if I caught it I'd know beyond any doubt, a person had only three days of fever in which to find out. Some had swellings behind their ears, some under their armpits, on their bellies, buboes developed, then a fever took over; sometimes the boils burst, sometimes blood spewed from the lungs, there were those who died violently like consumptives. He added that people from every district were dying in threes and fives. Anxious, I asked about our own neighborhood. Hadn't I heard? A bricklayer who quarreled with all the neighbors because their chickens were getting in through his wall, had died screaming with fever just one week ago. Only now did everyone realize that he'd died of the plague.

But I still didn't want to believe it; outside in the streets everything looked so normal, people passing by the window were so calm, I needed to find someone to share my alarm if I were to believe the plague was here. The next morning, when Hoja went to school, I flew out into the streets. I searched out the Italian converts I'd managed to meet during the eleven years I had spent here. One of them known by his new name Mustafa Reis, had left for the dockyards; the other, Osman Efendi, wouldn't let me in at first although I knocked at his door as if I would beat it down with my fists. He had his servant say he wasn't at home but finally gave in and shouted after me. How could I still question whether the disease was real; didn't I see those coffins carried down the street? He said I was scared, he could see it in my face, I was scared because I remained faithful to Christianity! He scolded me; a man must be a Muslim to be happy here, but he neglected to press my hand before he retreated into the dank darkness of his own house, didn't touch me at all. It was the hour of prayer, and when I saw the crowds in the courtyards of the mosques, I was seized with fear and started for home. I was overcome by the bewilderment that strikes people at times of disaster. It was as if I had lost my past, as though my memory had been drained, I was paralyzed. When I saw a group carrying a funeral bier through the streets of our neighborhood it completely unnerved me.

Hoja had come back from the school, I sensed he was pleased when he saw how I was. I noticed that my fear increased his self-confidence and this made me uneasy. I wanted him to be rid of the vain pride in his fearlessness. Trying to check my agitation, I poured out all my medical and literary knowledge, I described what I remembered from the scenes of plague in Hippocrates, Thucydides and Boccacio, said it was believed the disease was contagious, but this only made him more contemptuous – he didn't fear the plague; disease was God's will, if a man was fated to die he would die; for this reason it was useless to talk cowardly nonsense as I did about shutting oneself up in one's house and severing relations with the outside or trying to escape from Istanbul. If it was written, so it would come to pass, death would find us. Why was afraid? Because of those sins of mine I'd written day by day? He smiled, his eyes shining with certainty.

Until the day we lost one another I was never able to find out if he really believed what he said. Seeing him so completely undaunted I had been afraid for a moment, but then, when I remembered our discussions at the table, those terrifying games he played, I became skeptical. He was circling around, steering the conversation to the sins we'd written down together. Reiterating the same idea with an air of conceit that drove me wild: if I was so afraid of death I couldn't have mastered the wickedness I appeared to write about so bravely. The courage I showed in pouring out my sins was simply the result my shamelessness! Whereas he hesitated at the time because he was so painstakingly attentive to the tiniest fault. But now he was calm, the deep confidence he felt in the face of the plague had left no doubt in his heart that he must be innocent.

Repelled by this explanation, which I stupidly believed, I decided to argue with him. Naively I suggested that he was confident not he had a clear conscience but because he did not know that death was so near. I explained how we could protect ourselves from death, that we must not touch those who had caught the plague, the corpses must be buried in limed pits, that people must reduce their contact with one another as much as possible, and that Hoja must not go that crowded school.

It seems that this last thing I said gave him ideas even more horrible than plague. The next day at noon, saying he'd touched each of the children at school one by one, he stretched out his hands towards me; when he saw me balk, that I was afraid to touch him, he came closer and embraced me with glee; I wanted to scream, but like someone in a dream, I couldn't cry out. As for Hoja, he said, with a derisiveness I only learned to understand much later, that he was going to teach me fearlessness.

The Old Doctor (*from* Cancer Ward)

Alexander Solzhenitsyn

In his seventy-five years of life and half century of treating disease Dr. Oreshchenkov had raised himself no stone mansion, but he had bought himself, back in the twenties, a one-story wooden house with a small garden. He had lived in it ever since. The little house stood in one of the quiet streets, a wide boulevard with a spacious sidewalk which put a good fifteen meters between the street and the houses. Back in the last century, trees with thick trunks had taken root in the pavement. In the summertime their tops met to make a continuous green roof. The base of each tree was dug round, cleared and protected by a neat cast-iron grill.

However scorching the sun, the people walking along the sidewalk felt none of its severity. Cool irrigation water ran along in a tiled ditch. This arch-shaped street ran round the most solid, attractive part of town, and was itself one of the town's finest adornments. (However, the town council grumbled that these one-story houses weren't close enough together, and this made the public utility models too expensive. It was time to pull them down and build five-story apartment blocks.)

The bus did not stop near Oreshchenkov's house, so Ludmila Afanasyevna went there on foot. It was a very warm evening, dry and not yet twilight, and she could see the trees preparing themselves for the night. The first tender fuzz of leaves had appeared on their branches, denser on some, thinner on others, while there was as yet no green at all in the candle-shaped poplars. But Dontsova was looking not upward but down at her feet. This year spring brought her no joy. Joy had been suspended as far as she was concerned, and no one knew what was going to hap-pen to Ludmila Afanasyevna while all these trees were breaking into leaf, and while the leaves turned yellow and were finally shed. Even before her illness she'd been so busy the whole time that she'd never had a chance to stop, throw back her head, crinkle her eyes and look upward.

Dr. Oreshchenkov's house was guarded by a wooden-slatted door, alongside which stood an old-fashioned front door with a brass handle and heavy pyramid-shaped panels. In houses like these the old doors were usually nailed up and one entered by the new door. But here the two stone steps that led up to the old door were not overgrown with grass and moss. There was a copper plate with sloping calligraph-ic writing on it. "Dr. D. T. Oreshchenkov" it read, and it was polished as brightly as it had been in the old days. The electric bell was set in a little cup. It did not look unused.

Ludmila Afanasyevna pressed the button. She heard a few steps and the door was opened by Oreshchenkov himself. He had on a well-worn brown suit (it had once been a good one) and an open-necked shirt.

"Aha, Ludochka!" he said, raising the corners of his lips slightly. But with him this was the broadest of smiles. "Come in, I've been waiting, I'm very glad to see you. I'm glad, but I'm also not glad. You wouldn't come visiting an old man if it was something good."

She had telephoned him and asked permission to call. She could have told him what it was about on the telephone, but that wouldn't have been very polite. She was now guiltily trying to convince him that she would have called anyway, even if she hadn't been in trouble, while he was refusing to let her take off her coat by herself. "Please, allow me," he said. "I'm not an old ruin yet."

He hung her coat on one of the pegs of a long, dark, polished coat rack ready to receive any number of guests or visitors, and led her across the smoothly painted wooden floor. The corridor took them past the best and brightest room in the house. In it was a grand piano with a raised music stand, the pages of the score open and gay-looking. It was here that Oreshchenkov's eldest granddaughter lived. They walked across into the dining room. It had windows draped with dry grapevines and giving out onto the yard. In the room was a large and expensive radio-phonograph. After this they came to the consulting room, which had walls lined with bookshelves, a heavy old-fashioned writing desk, an old sofa and some comfortable armchairs.

"Well, Dormidont Tikhonovich," said Dontsova, gazing round the wall and narrowing her eyes. "It looks as though you've got even more books than before."

"Oh no, not really," Oreshchenkov replied, shaking his head fractionally. His head seemed to have been cast out of metal. He shook it very slightly; all his gestures were slight. "Oh, it's true, I did buy a couple of dozen lately, and you know who from?" He looked at her merrily, just a shade merrily; you had to know him to notice all these nuances. "I got them from Kaznacheyev. He's retired, he's just turned sixty, you know. And on the actual day of his retirement it turned out he wasn't a radiologist at heart at all, he didn't want to spend another day of his life on medicine. He'd always wanted to be a beekeeper, and now bees are the only thing he'll take an interest in. How do these things happen, do you think? If you're really a beekeeper, how is it that you waste the best years of your life doing something else? Well now, where would you like to sit, Ludochka?" She was a grand-mother with graying hair, but he spoke to her as he would to a little girl. He made up her mind for her. "Take this armchair, you'll be comfortable here."

"I won't stay long, Dormidont Tikhonovich, I only dropped in for a minute," said Dontsova, still protesting, but by now she had sunk deep into a soft armchair. Immediately she felt calm. She felt almost confident that in this room only the best possible decisions could be taken. The burden of permanent responsibility, the burden of administration, the burden of choosing what she ought to do with her life, had been lifted from her shoulders at the coat rack in the corridor. Now she was deep in the armchair her problems had finally collapsed. Calm and relaxed, she let her eyes travel slowly round the room which, of course, she knew of old. It touched her to see the old marble washstand basin in the corner, not a modern washbasin but one with a bucket underneath it. It was all covered, though, and very clean.

She looked straight at Oreshchenkov, glad that he was alive, that he was there and would take all her anxiety upon himself. He was still on his feet. He stood upright without the faintest stoop, shoulders and head set as firmly as ever. He always had this look of confidence. It was as though, while he treated other people, he was absolutely sure he could never fall ill himself. A small, neatly cut silvery beard streamed from the middle of his chin. His head was not yet bald, not even com-pletely gray, and the smooth part of his hair seemed to have changed hardly at all over the years. He had the kind of face whose features are not moved by emotion. Every line remained smooth, calm and in place, except for his habit of raising his eyebrows almost imperceptibly into archlike angles. Only his eyebrows expressed the full range of his emotions.

"If you'll forgive me, Ludochka," he said, "I'll sit at the desk. It's not that I want it to look like a formal interview, it's just that I'm used to sitting there."

It would be a miracle if he hadn't been. It was to this room that his patients had always come, frequently at first, almost every day, then more rarely. But they still came, even now. Sometimes they would sit through long, painful conversations on which their whole future depended. As the conversation twisted and turned, the green baize of the table, outlined by the margins of dark-brown oak, might engrave itself on their memories for the rest of their lives. So might the old wood-en paperknife, the nickel-plated spatula which helped him see down throats, the flipover calendar, the inkpot under its copper lid, or the very strong tea he drank—the color of deep claret—which grew cold in the glass. The doctor would sit at his desk, occasionally getting up and walking toward the washstand or the bookshelves to give the patient a chance to relax from his gaze and to think things over. Dr. Oreshchenkov would never look to one side without good reason. His eyes reflected the constant attention he gave both patient and visitor; they never missed a moment for observation, never wandered toward the window or stared down at the desk or the papers on it. His eyes were the chief instrument he used to study his patients and students, to convey his decisions or wishes.

Dormidont Tikhonovich had suffered from persecution several times during his life: for revolutionary activities in 1902 when he and some other students spent a week or so in jail; again, because his late father had been a priest; then for having been a brigade medical officer in the Tsarist army during the First Imperialist War. (It was not just because he'd been a medical officer; according to the testimony of witnesses, he had mounted a horse while his regiment was in panic retreat, rallied the regiment and dragged it back to take part in the imperialist slaughter of German workers.) The most persistent and oppressive persecution had been due to his stubborn insistence on his right to maintain a private medical practice in the face of stricter and stricter prohibitions. What he did was forbidden as a source of private enterprise and enrichment, as an activity, divorced from honest labor, that served as a daily breeding ground for the bourgeoisie. There were years when he had had to take down his copper plate and turn away every patient, no matter how much they implored him or how ill they were. This was because the neighborhood was full of spies from the tax office, paid or voluntary, and because the patients themselves could never refrain from talking. As a result, the doctor was threatened with the loss of all work, even with the loss of his house.

But it was precisely this right to run a private practice that he valued most in his profession. Without the engraved plate on the door he lived as if illegally or under an assumed name. He refused to submit either his Master's or Doctor's thesis as a matter of principle, on the ground that a thesis was no indication whatever of the success of day-to-day treatment, that it made a patient uneasy having a doctor who was a professor, and that the time spent on the thesis could be much more usefully spent picking up an extra branch of medicine. During Oreshchenkov's thirty years at the local medical college, quite apart from his other jobs, he had helped provide general treatment and also worked in the pediatric, surgical, epidemic, urological and even ophthalmological clinics. It was only after all this that he became a radiologist and oncologist. He would employ a one-millimeter compression of the lips to express his opinion about "Honored Scientists." He claimed that if a man was called a "Scientist" during his lifetime, and an "Honored" one at that, it was the end of him as a doctor. The honor and glory of it all would get in the way of his treatment of his patients just as elaborate clothing hinders a man's movements. These "Honored Scientists" went about with a suite of followers, like some new Christ with his Apostles. They completely lost the right to make mistakes or not to know something, they lost the right to be allowed to think things over. The man might be self-satisfied, half-witted, behind the times, and trying to conceal the fact, and yet everyone would expect miracles from him.

Oreshchenkov wanted none of this sort of thing for himself. All he needed was a brass plate on his door and a bell which any passer-by could ring.

Luckily for him, Oreshchenkov had once happened to save a local VIP's son who was at death's door. On a different occasion he had saved another big shot, not the same one but a very important person nevertheless. There were several members of other important families as well who owed their lives to him. It had all taken place here in the one town, since he had never gone away. As a result, Dr. Oreshchenkov's reputation became established in influential circles and a certain aura of protection was built up around him. In a purely Russian city this might well not have helped, but the East was more easygoing and they were willing to overlook the fact that he had hung up his plate and was accepting patients again. After the war he no longer held a regular permanent appointment, but served as consultant in several clinics and attended meetings of scientific societies. So it was that after the age of sixty-five he began to lead the sort of unhindered life he regarded as right for a doctor.

"So, Dormidont Tikhonovich, I came to ask you to come down and give me a gastrointestinal examination. Any day that suits you, we'll arrange it."

She looked gray and her voice faltered. Oreshchenkov watched her steadily, his glance never wavering and his angular eyebrows expressing not one millimeter of surprise.

"Of course, Ludmila Afanasyevna. We shall arrange the day. However, I should like you to explain what your symptoms are, and what you think about them yourself."

"I'll tell you my symptoms right away, but as for what I think about them—well, you know, I try not to think about them. That is to say, I think about them all too much, and now I've begun not sleeping at nights. The best thing would be if I knew nothing. I'm serious! You decide whether I'm to go into hospital or not and I'll go, but I don't want to know the details. If I'm to have an operation I would rather not know the diagnosis, otherwise I'll be thinking the whole time during the operation, 'What on earth are they doing to me now? What are they taking out now?' Do you understand?"

Whether it was the size of the armchair or the way her shoulders sagged, somehow she no longer looked a big, strong woman. She had shrunk.

"Understand? Well, perhaps I do understand, Ludochka, but I don't share your opinion. Anyway, why is an operation your first thought?"

"Well, we have to be ready for…"

"Why didn't you come here earlier, then? You of all people?"

"Well, you see, Dormidont Tikhonovich…" Dontsova sighed. "That's the way life is, one whirl after another. Of course I should've come earlier…But you mustn't think I've let it go too far." She was protesting vigorously more to herself than to anyone else. She had regained her brisk, businesslike way of talking. "Why does it have to be so unjust? Why should I, an oncologist, be struck down by an oncological disease, when I know every single one of them, when I can imagine all the attendant effects, consequences and complications?"

"There's no injustice there," he replied. His bass voice was measured and very persuasive. "On the contrary, it is justice in the highest degree. It's the truest of all tests for a doctor to suffer from the disease he specializes in."

(What's just about it? Why is it such a true test? He only talks like this because he's not ill himself.)

"Do you remember that nurse Panya Fyodorova?" he continued. "She used to say, 'Oh dear, why am I being so rude to the patients? It's time I went in as a patient again…' "

"I never thought I'd take it so hard," said Dontsova, cracking her interlocked fingers.

Yet in these few minutes she had felt much less anguish than during recent weeks.

"So what have you observed in the way of symptoms?"

She began to tell him in general outline, but he wanted to know the precise details.

"Dormidont Tikhonovich, the last thing I want to do is to take up the whole of your Saturday evening. If you're coming to give me an X-ray examination anyway…"

"Well, you know what a heretic I am, don't you? You know I worked for twenty years before X rays were invented. And, my dear, you should have seen the diagnoses I made! It's like when you have an exposure meter or a watch, you completely lose the knack of estimating exposure by eye or judging time by instinct. When you don't have them, you soon acquire the trick."

Dontsova began to explain, grouping and differentiating the symptoms and forcing herself not to omit any details which might point toward a crushing diagnosis. (But in spite of herself she was tempted to omit some of them, just to hear him say, "It's nothing serious, Ludochka, it's nothing at all.") She told him her blood composition, which wasn't at all good, and her blood count, which was too high. At first he listened to her without interrupting, then he asked her some questions. Sometimes he nodded his head to indicate that something was readily understandable and frequently encountered, but he never said "It's nothing." The thought flashed through Dontsova's mind that he must have made his diagnosis already, that she might as well ask him straight out without waiting for the X ray. But it was terrifying, the idea of asking him here and now and getting an answer, whether correct or incorrect or even tentative. She had to put it off, she had to soften the blow by a few days of waiting.

They talked as friends talk when they meet at a scientific conference. Yet having confessed to being ill was like having confessed to a crime: immediately they had lost the key to the equality they had once possessed. No, perhaps not equality; there had never been equality between her and her teacher. It was more drastic than that. By her confession she had excluded herself from the noble estate of medical men and transferred herself to the taxpaying, dependent estate of patients.

It was true that Oreshchenkov did not at once ask if he could feel where it hurt her. He continued to talk to her as to a guest. He seemed to be inviting her to join both estates at once. But she had been crushed, she had lost her former bearing.

"Quite frankly, Verochka Gangart is such a good diagnostician now that I'd normally have had complete confidence in her," said Dontsova, firing out sentences in the rapid manner her crowded working day forced her to adopt. "But it's you, Dormidont Tikhonovich, I thought I'd…"

"I'd be a fine one if I turned down my own students," Oreshchenkov replied, looking at her steadily. Dontsova couldn't see him very well at the moment, but for the last two years she'd noticed a certain gleam of detachment in his unswerving gaze. It had appeared after the death of his wife. "But if you have to…take sick leave for a bit, will Verochka take your place?"

(Take sick leave! He had chosen the mildest term of all! Did it mean, did it mean there was nothing wrong with her?)

Yes, she will. She's a mature specialist now, she's quite capable of running the department."

Oreshchenkov nodded. He gripped his narrow beard. "Yes," he said, "she may be a mature specialist, but what about her getting married?"

Dontsova shook her head.

My granddaughter's like that too," Oreshchenkov went on, his voice dropping to a whisper, quite unnecessarily. "She can't find anyone right for her. It's a difficult business."

The angles of his eyebrows shifted slightly to register his concern.

He made a point of insisting there should be no delay. He would examine Dontsova on Monday.

(Why was he in such a hurry?...)

Then came the pause when, presumably, it was time for her to say "Thank you" and take her leave. She stood up, but Oreshchenkov insisted she take a glass of tea with him.

"Really, I don't want any tea," Ludmila Afanasyevna told him.

"Well, I do. It's just time for my tea." He was making a determined effort to pull her out of the category of the criminally ill into the category of the hopelessly healthy.

"Are your young people at home?" she asked him.

The young people were the same age as Ludmila Afanasyevna.

"No, they're not. My granddaughter isn't here either. I'm on my own."

(Still, it was in his consulting room that he had received her as a doctor. It was only here that he could impress her with the true significance of what he said.)

"Are you going to play the hostess for me, then?" she said. "Because I won't let you."

"No, there's no need for that. I've got a full thermos. There are some cakes and plates for them in the cupboard; you can get them if you like."

They moved into the dining room and sat down to drink their tea at one corner of a square oak table, big enough for an elephant to dance on and much too big to be got through any of the doors. The wall clock, not in its first youth, showed that it was still quite early.

***

…He had noticed the momentary troubled, confused, impatient expression on Dontsova's face. But since she wasn't eager to know the nature of her disease, why keep going over the symptoms on Saturday night when she would only have to step behind an X-ray machine on Monday? It was his job to distract her by conversation, and what better topic could there be for doctors to talk about? "Generally speaking," he remarked, "the family doctor is the most comforting figure in our lives, and now he's being pulled up by the roots. The family doctor is a figure without whom the family cannot exist in a developed society. He knows the needs of each member of the family, just as the mother knows their tastes. There's no shame in taking to him some trivial complaint you'd never take to the outpatients' clinic, which entails getting an appointment card and waiting your turn, and where there's a quota of nine patients an hour. And yet all neglected illnesses arise out of these trifling complaints. How many adult human beings are there, now, at this minute, rushing about in mute panic wishing they could find a doctor, the kind of person to whom they can pour out the fears they have deeply concealed or even found shameful? Looking for the right doctor is the sort of thing you can't always ask your friends for advice about. You can't advertise for one in a newspaper either. In fact, it's a matter as essentially intimate as a search for a husband or a wife. But nowadays it's easier to find a good wife than a doctor ready to look after you personally for as long as you want, and who understands you fully and truly."

Ludmila Afanasyevna frowned. These were abstract ideas. Meanwhile her head was whirling with more and more symptoms arranging themselves in the worst possible pattern.

"That's all very well, but how many family doctors would you need? It simply doesn't fit into the system of a free universal national health service."

"It'll fit into a universal national health service, but it won't fit into a free health service," said Oreshchenkov, rumbling on and clinging confidently to his point.

"But it's our greatest achievement, the fact that it's a free service."

"Is this in fact such a great achievement? What does 'free' mean? The doctors don't work for nothing, you know. It only means that they're paid out of the national budget and the budget is supported by patients. It isn't free treatment, it's depersonalized treatment. If a patient kept the money that pays for his treatments, he would have turned the ten roubles he has to spend at the doctor's over and over in his hands. He could go to the doctor five times over if he really needed to."

"But he wouldn't be able to afford it?"

"He would say, 'To hell with the new drapes and spare pair of shoes. What's the use of them if I'm not healthy?' Is it any better as things are now? You would be ready to pay goodness knows how much for a decent reception at the doctor's, but there's no one to go to get it. They all have their schedules and their quotas, and so it's 'Next patient, please.' As for the clinics that do charge fees, the turnover's even faster than in the others. Why do people go there? Because they want a chit or certificate or sick leave or an invalid's pension card. The doctor's job there is to catch the malingerers; patients and doctors are like enemies. Do you call that medicine? Or take actual drugs and medicine, for instance. In the twenties all medicines were free. Do you remember?"

"Is that right? Yes, I think they were. One forgets."

"You'd really forgotten, have you? They were all free of charge, but we had to give it up. Do you know why?"

"I suppose it must have been too expensive for the government," said Dontsova with an effort, closing her eyes for a short while.

"It wasn't only that, it was also that it was extremely wasteful. The patient was bound to grab all the drugs he could since they cost him nothing and the result was he threw half of them away. Of course I'm not saying all treatments should be paid for by the patient. It's the primary treatment that ought to be. After a patient has been directed to enter hospital or undergo treatment that involves complicated apparatus, then it's only fair it should be free. But even so, take any clinic: why do two surgeons do the operations while the other three just gape at them? Because they get their salaries come what may, so why worry? If they got their money from the patients, nobody would ever consult them. Then your Halmuhamedov and your Pantyokhina would be running round in circles, wouldn't they? One way or the other, Ludochka, the doctor should depend on the impression he makes on his patients, he should be dependent on his popularity. Nowadays, he isn't."

"God help us if we had to depend on every single patient, that scandalmonger Polina Zavodchikova, for instance…"

"No, we should depend on her as well."

"That's sheer humiliation!"

"Is it any worse than depending on the senior doctor? Is it any less honest than drawing a government salary like some bureaucratic civil servant?"

"But some of these patients dig down into every detail—Rabinovich and Kostoglotov, for example. They wear you out asking theoretical questions. Are we supposed to answer every single one?"

Not a crease furrowed Oreshchenkov's high forehead. He had always known Ludmila Dontsova's limitations: they were not narrow, either. She was quite capable of considering and treating the trickiest cases, all on her own as well. The two hundred or so unassuming little items she had published in medical journals were examples of the most difficult type of diagnosis, which was the most difficult aspect of medicine. Why should he expect any more of her?

"That's right," he said, you must answer every single one."

"Well, where do we find the time?" objected Dontsova indignantly, warming up to the argument. It was all very well for him, walking up and down the room in his slippers. "Have you any idea what the pace of work is like at medical institutions nowadays? It was different in your day. Just think how many patients there are for every doctor."

"With the right kind of primary system," Oreshchenkov countered, "there'd be fewer cases altogether, and no neglected ones. The primary doctor should have no more patients than his memory and personal knowledge can cover. Then he could treat each patient as a subject on his own. Treating diseases separately is work on the feldsher level."

"Oh dear!" sighed Dontsova wearily. As if there was any chance of their private conversation changing or reforming anything of consequence! "It's a frightening thought, treating each patient as a subject on his own."

Oreshchenkov too sensed that it was time he stopped. Verbosity was a vice he had developed in his old age.

"But the patient's organism isn't aware that our knowledge is divided into separate branches. You see, the organism isn't divided. As Voltaire said, 'Doctors prescribe medicines about which they know little for an organism about which they know less.' How can we understand the patient as a single subject? After all, the anatomist who draws the charts operates on corpses; the living aren't his province, are they? A radiologist makes a name for himself on bone fractures; the gastrointestinal tract is outside his field, isn't it? The patient gets tossed from 'specialist' to 'specialist' like a basketball. That's why a doctor can remain a passionate beekeeper, all through his career. If you wanted to understand the patient as a single subject, there'd be no room left in you for any other passion. That's the way it is. The doctor should be a single subject as well. The doctor ought to be an all-rounder."

"The doctor as well?" It was almost a plaintive groan. If she'd been able to keep her spirits up and a clear head no doubt she would have found this exhaustive discussion interesting. But as things were they merely broke her morale even further. She found it so hard to concentrate.

"Yes, Ludochko, and you're just such a doctor. You shouldn't undersell yourself. There's nothing new about this, you know. Before the Revolution we municipal doctors all had to do it. We were clinical specialists, not administrators. Nowadays the senior doctor of a district hospital insists on having ten specialists on his staff, otherwise he won't work."

He could see it was time to finish. Ludmila Afanasyevna's exhausted face and blinking eyes showed that the conversation designed to distract her had done her no good at all. Just then the door from the veranda opened and in came…it looked like a dog but it was such a big, warm, unbelievable creature that it resembled even more a man who had for some reason gone down on all fours. Ludmila Afanasyevna's first impulse was to be afraid he might bite her, but one could no more be afraid of him than of an intelligent, sad-eyed human being.

He moved across the room softly, almost as though he were deep in thought, without the faintest inkling that anyone in the house might be surprised at his entrance. He raised his luxuriant white brush of a tail, waved it once to say hello and lowered it. Apart from two black drooping ears he was ginger-white, two colors alternating in his fur in a complicated pattern. On his back he was wearing what looked like a white horse blanket, but his sides were bright ginger and his rear almost orange. True, he did come up to Ludmila Afanasyevna and sniff her knees, but he did it quite unobtrusively. He did not sit down on his orange hindquarters next to the table as one would expect a dog to do. He expressed no interest in the food on the table just above the top of his head. All he did was stand there on all fours, his great liquid-brown eyes peering up over the edge of the table in transcendental detachment.

"Good heavens, what breed's that?" Ludmila Afanasyevna was so amazed that for the first time that evening she had completely forgotten herself and her pain.

"He's a Saint Bernard," replied Oreshchenkov, looking at the dog encouragingly. "He'd be all right except that his ears are too long. Manya gets furious when she feeds him. 'Shall I tie them up with string for you?' she says. 'They keep slopping into the dish!' "

Ludmila Afanasyevna inspected the dog and was struck with admiration. There was no place for such a dog in the bustle of the streets. They'd never allow a dog like that onto public transport. If the Himalayas were the only place left where an abominable snowman could live, the only place for this dog was the garden of a one-story house.

Oreshchenkov cut a slice of cake and offered it to the dog. But he didn't throw it to him as one throws things for fun or out of pity to other sorts of dogs, to see them stand on their hind legs or jump up, teeth chattering. If this one stood on his hind legs it would not be to beg, but to put his paws on human shoulders as a sign of friendship. Oreshchenkov offered him the cake as an equal, and he took it as an equal, his teeth calmly and unhurriedly removing it from the doctor's palm as though from a plate. He might not even have been hungry; he might have taken it out of politeness.

The arrival of this tranquil, thoughtful dog somehow refreshed Ludmila Afanasyevna and cheered her up. She rose from the table thinking that maybe she wasn't in such a bad state after all, even if she did have to undergo an operation. She hadn't been paying Dormidont Tikhonovich enough attention, though.

"I've become absolutely unscrupulous," she said. "I've come here bringing you all my aches and pains and I haven't even asked how you are. How are you?"

He stood facing her, straightbacked, on the portly side; his eyes had not yet begun to water; his ears could hear every sound. It was impossible to believe he was twenty-five years older than she was.

"All right so far," he said smiling. It was an amiable smile but not a very warm one. "I've decided I'm never going to be ill before I die. I'll just give up the ghost, as they say."

He saw her out, came back into the dining room and sank into a rocking chair of black bentwood and yellow wickerwork, its back worn by the years he had spent in it. He gave it a pushoff as he sat and let the movement die down. He did not rock it any more. He was sitting in the odd position peculiar to rocking chairs. It was almost off balance but free. He froze like that for a long time, completely motionless.

He had to take frequent rests nowadays. His body demanded this chance to recoup its strength and with the same urgency his inner self demanded silent contemplation free of external sounds, conversations, thoughts of work, free of everything that made him a doctor. Particularly after the death of his wife, his inner consciousness had seemed to crave a pure transparency. It was just this sort of silent immobility, without planned or even floating thoughts, which gave him a sense of purity and fulfillment.

At such moments an image of the whole meaning of existence—his own during the long past and the short future ahead, that of his late wife, of his young granddaughter and of everyone in the world—came to his mind. The image he saw did not seem to be embodied in the work or activity which occupied them, which they believed was central to their lives, and by which they were known to others. The meaning of existence was to preserve unspoiled, undisturbed and undistorted the image of eternity with which each person is born.

Like a silver moon in a calm, still pond.

from A Whole New Life: An Illness and a Healing

Reynolds Price

Was it disaster—all that time from my slapped-down sandal in spring '84 through the four years till I reentered life as a new contraption, inside and out? Is it still disaster, these ten years later? Numerous mouths and pairs of eyes have been, and still are, ready to tell me Yes every week. Very often occasional acquaintances will corner me on campus or at a party, then lean to my ear and ask how I am. When I tell them truthfully "Fine," their faces will crouch in solemn concern; and they'll say "No, really. How are you?" I'll give them a skull-grin to cover my amusement at the common eagerness of so many otherwise decent souls to see a fellow creature buried.

My amusement flows also from their hint that they know I'm hoarding a tragic secret to which they have an intimate right. They plainly believe that any chink in the normal human armor is a road down which all the curious are free to stream. That brand of assault is especially common now in politically correct middle-class America where the socially and physically gimped are crowned with a misplaced, thoroughly unwanted beatitude—the blessings of sainthood are mostly appalling as they've always been.

Physicians, in their admirable Greek and Latin mode, speak of a "catastrophic" illness. The Greek word catastrophe means an overturning, an upending—a system disarranged past reassembly, all signals reversed. The list of common catastrophes that wait for a final chance at each of us is virtually endless; and it now receives unimagined additions almost by the week from a viral kingdom that begins to hint at the chance of its ultimate victory over us, through cunning and patience.

Birth disasters, unstoppable cancers, disorders of the blood and lymph, external wounds to flesh and bone, those devastations in which the body turns on itself and eats its own substance, the mind's estrangement, the still irreparable disconnection of electrical service to major parts—each of a throng of catastrophes is as common as influenza or migraine, and so far I've missed a great many blows aimed at me; but I took this big one.

So disaster then, yes, for me for a while—great chunks of four years. Catastrophe surely, a literally upended life with all parts strewn and some of the most urgent parts lost for good, within and without. But if I were called on to value honestly my present life beside my past—the years from 1933 till '84 against the years after—I'd have to say that, despite an enjoyable fifty-year start, these recent years since full catastrophe have gone still better. They've brought more in and sent more out—more love and care, more knowledge and patience, more work in less time.

How self-deluding, self-serving, is that? Why do physically damaged people so often meet the world with clear bright eyes and what seem unjustified or lunatic smiles? Have some few layers of our minds burned off, leaving us dulled to the shocks of life, the actual state of our devastation? Or are we merely displaying a normal animal pleasure in being at least alive and breathing, not outward bound to the dark unknown or anxious for some illusory safety, some guarantee we know to be ludicrous?

Maybe I'd answer a partial Yes to all such questions. Though there's no "we" of course in the damaged world—the possible array of damage is too vast—I can risk a few observations at least that have proved true for me, through much of the time, and that may prove useful to someone else who's faced with a sudden blank wall in life and who may care to hear them, for companionship if nothing more.

I take the risk for one main reason that I've mentioned earlier—friends and strangers have asked me to add my recollections to the very slim row of sane printed matter which comes from the far side of catastrophe, the dim other side of that high wall that effectively shuts disaster off from the unfazed world. I've known what they mean. I shared their frustration for some fellow-words to consume in those weeks after radiation in '84 when I finally recovered the will to read and searched around me for any book, essay or sentence that might speak directly to the hole I was in—anything more useful than crackpot guides to healing or death, impossibly complex starvation diets, alfalfa pills and karmic tune-ups. In that deep trough I needed companions more than prayers or potions that had worked for another. But nothing turned up in my own library, apart from short stretches of the Bible, or in all the would-be helpful books that friends sent to me on every subject from crystals and macrobiotic cooking through cheerful wheel-chair tours of Europe and the rules for a last will and testament.

Most of the books were either telling me why I had cancer—the utterly unproved claim again that I'd somehow brought it home in self-loathing—or they blithely prescribed in minute detail how to cure any tumor with moon-rock dust and bee-tle-wing ointment. Or they cheerfully told me what kind of deal I should offer God in hopes of the maximum chance at salvage—I give you two good legs, the power of feeling from the soles of my feet on up to my nipples, control of numerous internal organs, and acceptance of pain like an acid bath with no letup. For that, you'll kindly permit me to crawl in and gorge my face by the television for however many minutes or years you can spare from your big store of eternity.

I needed to read some story that paralleled, at whatever distance, my unfolding bafflement—some honest report from a similar war, with a final list of hard facts learned and offered unvarnished—but again I never found it. Admitted, there are richly useful methods, like the twelve-step program of Alcoholics Anonymous, for reversing long years of self-abuse. And the scathing self-disciplines of some religious sects have turned weak souls into flaming martyrs singing in the yawning teeth of Hell. But nobody known to me in America, or on the shady backside of Pluto, is presently offering useful instruction in how to absorb the staggering but not-quite-lethal blow of a fist that ends your former life and offers you nothing by way of a new life that you can begin to think of wanting, though you clearly have to go on feeding your gimped-up body and roofing the space above your bed.

So after ten years at what seems a job that means to last me till death at least, I'll offer a few suggestions from my own slow and blundering course. I make no claim for their wisdom or even their usefulness. Whether they'll prove merely private to me or available to a handful of others as ground for thought, I'd likely be the last to know; but at least I can try to keep them honest. Here then are the minimal facts that eventually worked for me, at least part of the time, and are working still. In all that follows, the pronoun You is aimed at me as much as any reader. I need steady coaching; I'm never home-free. And when I refer to physical paralysis, I often suspect that other kinds of mind and body paralysis bring similar troubles with similar remedies.

Fairly late in the catastrophic phase of my illness, I began to understand three facts I'd known in theory since early childhood but had barely plumbed the reality of. They're things familiar to most adults who've bothered to watch the visible world and have sorted their findings with normal intelligence, but abstract knowledge tends to vanish in a crisis. And from where I've been, the three facts stand at the head of any advice I'd risk conveying to a friend confronted with grave illness or other physical and psychic trauma.

You're in your present calamity alone, far as this life goes. If you want a way out, then dig it yourself, if there turns out to be any trace of a way. Nobody—least of all a doctor—can rescue you now, not from the deeps of your own mind, not once they've stitched your gaping wound.

Generous people—true practical saints, some of them boring as root canals—are waiting to give you everything on Earth but your main want, which is simply the person you used to be.

But you're not that person now. Who'll you be tomorrow? And who do you propose to be from here to the grave, which may be hours or decades down the road?

The first two facts take care of themselves; if you haven't already known them in spades and obeyed their demands, they'll blow you nearly down till you concede their force. Harder though, and even more urgent, admit the third fact as soon as you can. No child of the doomed Romanov czar, awaiting rescue or brutal death in 1917, was more firmly banished from a former life than you are now. Grieve for a decent limited time over what parts of your old self you know you'll miss.

That person is dead as any teenaged Marine drilled through the forehead in an Asian jungle; any Navy Seal with his legs blown off, halved for the rest of the time he gets; any woman mangled in her tenderest parts, unwived, unmothered, unlovered and shorn. Have one hard cry, if the tears will come. Then stanch the grief, by whatever legal means. Next find your way to be somebody else, the next viable you—a stripped-down whole other clear-eyed person, realistic as a sawed-off shotgun and thankful for air, not to speak of the human kindness you'll meet if you get normal luck.

Your mate, your children, your friends at work—anyone who knew or loved you in your old life—will be hard at work in the fierce endeavor to revive your old self, the self they recall with love or respect. Their motives are frequently admirable, and at times that effort counts for a lot—they prove that you're valued and wanted at least—but again their care is often a brake on the way you must go. At the crucial juncture, when you turn toward the future, they'll likely have little help to offer; and it's no fault of theirs (they were trained like you, in inertia).

More likely they'll stall you in the effort to learn who you need to be now and how to be him or her by tomorrow or Monday at the latest. Yet if you don't discover that next appropriate incarnation of who you must be, and then become that person at a stiff trot, you'll be no good whatever again to the ruins of your old self nor to any friend or mate who's standing beside you in hopes of a hint that you're feeling better this instant and are glad of company.

The kindest thing anyone could have done for me, once I'd finished five weeks' radiation, would have been to look me square in the eye and say this clearly, "Reynolds Price is dead. Who will you be now? Who can you be and how can you get there, double-time?" Cruel and unusable as it might have sounded in the wake of trauma, I think its truth would have snagged deep in me and won my attention eventually, far sooner than I managed to find it myself. Yet to this day, with all the kindnesses done for me, no one has so much as hinted that news in my direction; and I've yet to meet another dazed person who's heard it when it was needed most—Come back to life, whoever you'll be. Only you can do it.

How you'll manage that huge transformation is your problem though and nobody else's. Are there known techniques for surviving a literal hairpin turn in the midst of a life span—or early or late—without forgetting the better parts of who you were? What are the thoughts and acts required to turn your dead self inside-out into something new and durably practical that, however strange, is the creature demanded by whatever hard facts confront you now? So far as I've heard, nobody else knows—or knows in a way they can transfer to others. If they know, I haven't encountered their method. I'll go on sketching my own course then.

I've made it clear that the first strong props beneath my own collapse were prayer, a single vision that offered me healing, the one word More when I asked "What now?" and a frail continuing sense of purpose, though my hungry self often worked to drown any voice that might otherwise have reached me from the mind of God or plain common sense. But I well understand how that kind of help is all but incommunicable to anyone else not so inclined from childhood. If belief in an ultimately benign creator who notices his creatures is available to you, you may want to try at first to focus your will on the absolute first ground-level question to ask him, her or faceless it. Again, that's not "Why me?" but "What next?"

In general the human race has believed that a God exists who is at least partly good. Recent polls have shown that a huge majority of Americans pray in some form daily; even many self-defined atheists pray apparently. And thousands of years of testimony from sane men and women is serious evidence, if not full proof, that God may consult you in unannounced moments. If he does so at all, it will likely mean that you've taken prior pains to know him. He'll almost surely lurk beyond you in heavy drapery with face concealed. He's likewise announced, in most major creeds, his availability for fox-hole conversions. Yet foxhole occupants are often faced with his baffling slowness to answer calls, or they reach a perpetual busy signal or a cold-dead line. Again, the answer to most prayers is No.

My own luck here was long prepared, from early childhood; but as with all sorts of invisible luck, there have been forced treks these past ten years when I all but quit and begged to die. Even then though I'd try to recall a passage of daunting eloquence in the thirtieth chapter of the Book of Deuteronomy where the baffling God of Jews and Christians says

I call Heaven and Earth to witness against you today that I have set life and death in front of you, blessing and curse. Therefore choose life so that you and your seed may last to love the Lord your God ....

Clear as the offered choice is, such a reach for life is another tall order, especially for a human in agonized straits. But even if you omit the last phrase from God's proposition (that you last to love him, even if you're a confirmed disbeliever), you're still confronted with another iron fact. The visible laws of physical nature are willing you to last as long as you can. Down at the core, you almost certainly want to survive.

You're of course quite free to balk that wish, by killing yourself and ending your physical will to endure; but amazingly few pained people choose death by suicide. And fewer still consider the strangeness of their endless moaning when death is so easy. To be sure, either God or the laws of nature will eventually force you to fall and die. But that event can tend to itself, with slim help from you. Meanwhile whether you see yourself as the temporary home of a deathless soul or as the short-term compound of skin and bone called Homo sapiens, your known orders are simply to Live. Never give death a serious hearing till its ripeness forces your final attention and dignified nod. It will of course take you screaming if it must, if you insist.

And keep control of the air around you. Many well-meaning mates, lovers and friends will stand by, observing that you're in the throes of blind denial—Give up. Let go. Get them out of your sight and your hearing with red-hot haste; use whatever force or fury it takes. Then try to choose life. Then see who you can live with now.

In my case, life has meant steady work, work sent by God but borne on my own back and on the wide shoulders of friends who want me to go on living and have helped me with a minimum of tears and no sign of pity. My work admittedly has been of the sort that, when it's available, permits deep absorption. It's also brought me sufficient money to guarantee time for further work and appropriate space in which to do it. Since childhood I've been subject to frequent sixteen-hour days, chained to an easel or desk in my home and glad to be grounded. Some other home workers have similar luck—gardening, woodcraft, pottery, sewing, cooking, the ceaseless daily needs of a family. Even the man or woman who works in an office or mill, even at the dullest repetitive task, has a ready-made routine for muting painful cries from the self.

The killing dead-ends are strewn all around you in the idle or physically weak aftermath of calamity itself, the stunned hours of blank wall-gazing that eagerly await you. Find any legal way to avoid my first mistake, which was sitting still in cooperation with the cancer's will to finish me fast. Play cutthroat card games, leave the house when you can, go sit in the park near children at play, read to the children in a cancer ward, go donate whatever strength you've got to feeding the hungry or tending the millions worse off than you. I wish to God I had—any legal acts to break the inward gaze at my withering self.

As soon as I could walk after my first surgery, Allan Friedman urged me to make immediate plans to return to campus—put a cot in my office, go there daily, deal with the mail and at least see my colleagues for lunch and small talk, feel free to call on him anytime he kept clinic hours or to phone whenever. What he failed to know as a busy surgeon was, I'd never written ten words in my campus office and couldn't think of trying—I'd merely be alone in a different building. Since it was summer, most of my colleagues had fled their offices, unlike physicians who work all seasons; and Duke Hospital, as a place to visit, felt like sure death.

But now I know Friedman was more than half right. Professors were not my only colleagues; in the long years of my life at Duke, I'd built a sizable village of friends—members of the post-office staff, workers in the dining rooms, book-stores, librarians, campus cops. Any trip to campus would have involved my meeting their usual hardheaded cheer; I'd have heard their own tales of good and bad luck. (Not at all incidentally, one of my friends on the postal staff phoned me one Sunday, a few weeks into the ordeal, and said that the members of his church had just agreed—they'd bring me all my meals, five days a week. I was amazed and thanked them firmly but declined the offer, at least for then.)

Surely I should have forced myself to move outward from the menacing house far sooner than I did. Though I couldn't drive, and was years away from thinking of an appropriate car, I might at least have ridden with my friend Betsy Cox to her regular stints at a homeless shelter in downtown Durham. I could have made bologna sandwiches as fast as she and listened to stories harder than mine; and if I wet my pants in the process, well, who the hell hasn't? Couldn't I have gone out and learned some useful degree of proportion, setting my woes in the midst of the world, yet still have kept my silent hours for learning how much damage I'd taken and how to build on it?

Anyone for whom such recommendations seem overly rosy should not miss the point. Your chance of rescue from any despair lies, if it lies anywhere, in your eventual decision to abandon the deathwatch by the corpse of your old self and to search out a new inhabitable body. The old *Theologica Germanica* knew that "nothing burns in Hell but the self"—above all, the old self broiling in the fat of its endless self-pity.

By very slow inches, as I've said, the decision to change my life forced itself on me; and I moved ahead as if a path was actually there and would stretch on a while. As truly as I could manage here in an intimate memoir, without exposing the private gifts of men and women who never asked to perform in my books, I've tried to map the lines of that change and the ways I traveled toward the reinvention and reassembly of a life that bears some relations with a now-dead life but is radically altered, trimmed for a whole new wind and route. A different life and—till now at least, as again I've said—a markedly better way to live, for me and for my response to most of the people whom my life touches.

I've tested that word better for the stench of sentimentality, narcissism, blind optimism or lunacy. What kind of twisted fool, what megalomaniac bucking for canonization, would give his strong legs and control of a body that gave him fifty-one years' good service with enormous amounts of sensory pleasure (a body that played a sizable part in winning him steady love from others) and would then surrender normal control of a vigorous life in an ample house and far beyond it in exchange for what?—two legs that serve no purpose but ballast to a numb torso and the rest of a body that acts as a magnet to no one living, all soaked in corrosive constant pain?

I know that this new life is better for me, and for most of my friends and students as new, in two measurable ways. First, paraplegia with its maddening limitations has forced a degree of patience and consequent watchfulness on me, though as a writer I'd always been watchful. Shortly after my own paralysis, I heard two of Franklin Roosevelt's sons say that the primary change in their father, after polio struck him in mid-life and grounded him firmly, was an increased patience and a willingness to listen. If you doubt that patience must follow paralysis, try imagining that you can't escape whoever manages to cross your doorsill.

Forced to sit, denied the easy flight that legs provide, you either learn patience or you cut your throat, or you take up a bludgeon and silence whoever's in reach at the moment. As I survived the black frustration of so many new forms of powerlessness, I partly learned to sit and attend, to watch and taste whatever or whomever seemed likely or needy, far more closely than I had in five decades. The pool of human evidence that lies beneath my writing and teaching, if nothing more, has grown in the wake of that big change.

Then the slow migration of a sleepless and welcome sexuality from the center of my life to the cooler edge has contributed hugely to the increased speed and volume of my work, not to speak of the gradual resolution of hungers that—however precious to mind and body—had seemed past feeding. It's the sex that's moved, in fact, not the eros. The sense of some others as radiant and magnetic bodies, bodies that promise pleasure and good, is if anything larger in my life than before.

And especially now that my remaining senses are free from the heavy damper of methadone, all other pain drugs and the muscle relaxant baclofen that stunned me for seven years, specific desire does come again and find expression in new ways that match the rewards of the old. But the fact that, in ten years since the tumor was found, I've completed thirteen books—I'd published a first twelve in the previous twenty-two years—would seem at least another demonstration that human energy, without grave loss, may flow from one form into another and win the same consoling gains. (The question of why and how I was able to increase my rate is unanswerable, by me anyhow—a race with death and silence, a massive rerouting of sexual energy would be the easy answers. But if I was racing, I never felt chased; panic came elsewhere but never in my work. On the contrary, I sense strongly that the illness itself either unleashed a creature within me that had been restrained and let him run at his own hungry will; or it planted a whole new creature in place of the old.)

There've been other, maybe more private, gains. Once the hand wringers and ambulance chasers disperse from your side, you begin to feel and eventually savor the keener attentions of old friends who feel a complicated new duty to stand in closer. It's a duty that you have the duty to lighten, as Simone Weil said in her haunting law of friendship—

Our friends owe us what we think they will give us. We must forgive them this debt.

In a country as addicted to calamitous news as America now, word of your illness or imminent death will likely draw not just a ring of crows—not all of whom are eager to feed—but likewise a flock of serious watchers. Both halves of my written work, the books from 1962 to '84 and those thereafter, have benefited from new readers summoned by word of an ordeal survived, however briefly. When I traveled across the states in the spring of '92, following the publication of Blue Calhoun—twenty-three readings in fourteen cities—I caught for the first time in the eyes of strangers a certain intense eagerness of response that I doubt was won by my gray hair alone. A certified gimp, in working order, is often accorded an unearned awe which he may be forgiven for enjoying a moment till he rolls on past the nearest mirror and adjusts his vision for colder reality.

I'm left today, as I write this page, with an odd conclusion that's risky to state. But since it's not only thoroughly true but may well prove of use to another, I'll state it baldly—I've led a mainly happy life. I can safely push further. I've yet to watch another life that seems to have brought more pleasure to its owner than mine has to me. And that claim covers all my years except for the actual eye of the storm I've charted, from the spring of 1984 till fall '88.

I'm the son of brave magnanimous parents who'd have offered both legs in hostage for mine, if they'd been living when mine were required. I'm the brother of a laughing openhanded man with whom I've never exchanged an angry adult word nor wanted to. I'm the cousin of a woman who, with her husband, offered to see me through to the grave. I'm the neighbor of a couple who offered to share my life, however long I lasted. I'm the ward of a line of responsible assistants who've moved into my home and life at twelve-month intervals, taken charge of both the house and me and insured a safe and favorable atmosphere for ongoing work. I'm the friend of many more spacious and lively souls than I've earned. I've had, and still have, more love—in body and mind—than I dreamed of in my lone boyhood.

Doctors of superb craft and technical judgment, whatever their faults of attention and sympathy, ousted a lethal thing from my spine. Other resourceful attendants nursed me through pitch-black nights of roaring pain. An annual lot of intelligent students throws down a welcome gauntlet to me—Give us all you've got, no discount for pain. The unseen hand of the source of all has never felt absent as long as a week, and I share the sense of the holiday-painter as she finishes her canvas at the end of Virginia Woolf's To the Lighthouse—"I have had my vision." Mine was a vision of healing that's remained in force for a decade full, at the least, of work.

So though I travel for work and pleasure, here I sit most weeks at work toward the end of ten years rocked with threats and hair-breadth rescues. Though I make no forecast beyond today, annual scans have gone on showing my spine clear of cancer—clear of visible growing cells at least (few cancer veterans will boast of a "cure"). When Allan Friedman's physician-wife heard the story of my continuing recovery at my sixtieth-birthday party, she said to Allan "But that's miraculous." Allan faced her, grinned and said "You could say that."

I've long since weaned myself from all drugs but a small dose of antidepressant, an aspirin to thin my blood, an occasional scotch or a good red wine and a simple acid to brace my bladder against infection. I write six days a week, long days that often run till bedtime; and the books are different from what came before in more ways than age. I sleep long nights with few hard dreams, and now I've outlived both my parents. Even my handwriting looks very little like the script of the man I was in June of '84. Cranky as it is, it's taller, more legible, with more air and stride. It comes down the arm of a grateful man.

Defining a Doctor,
With a Tear, a Shrug and a Schedule

Abigail Zuger

I had two interns to supervise that month, and the minute they sat down for our first meeting, I sensed how the month would unfold.

The man's white coat was immaculate, its pockets empty save for a sleek Palm Pilot that contained his list of patients.

The woman used a large loose-leaf notebook instead, every dog-eared page full of lists of things to do and check, consultants to call, questions to ask. Her pockets were stuffed, and whenever she sat down, little handbooks of drug doses, wadded phone messages, pens, highlighters and tourniquets spilled onto the floor.

The man worked the hours legally mandated by the state, not a minute more, and sometimes considerably less. He was seldom in the hospital before 8 in the morning, and left by 5 unless he was on call. He ate a leisurely lunch every day and was never late for rounds.

The woman got to the hospital around dawn and was on the move for the rest of the day. Sometimes she went home when she was supposed to, but sometimes, if one of her patients was particularly sick, she would sign out to the covering intern and keep working, often talking to patients' relatives long into the night.

"I am now breaking the law," she would announce cheerfully to no one in particular, then trot off to do just a few final chores.

The man had a strict definition of what it meant to be a doctor. He did not, for instance, "do nurses' work" (his phrase). When one of his patients needed a specimen sent to the lab and the nurse didn't get around to it, neither did he. No matter how important the job was, no matter how hard I pressed him, he never gave in. If I spoke sternly to him, he would turn around and speak just as sternly to the nurse.

The woman did everyone's work. She would weigh her patients if necessary (nurses' work), feed them (aides' work), find salt-free pickles for them (dietitians' work) and wheel them to X-ray (transporters' work).

The man was cheerful, serene and well rested. The woman was overtired, hyperemotional and constantly late. The man was interested in his patients, but they never kept him up at night. The woman occasionally called the hospital from home to check on hers. The man played tennis on his days off. The woman read medical articles. At least, she read the beginnings; she tended to fall asleep halfway through.

I felt as if I was in a medieval morality play that month, living with two costumed symbols of opposing philosophies in medical education. The woman was working the way interns used to: total immersion seasoned with exhaustion and adrenaline. As far as she was concerned, her patients were her exclusive responsibility. The man was an intern of the new millennium. His hours and duties were delimited; he saw himself as part of a health care team, and his patients' welfare as a shared responsibility.

This new model of medical internship got some important validation in The New England Journal of Medicine last week, when Harvard researchers reported the effects of reducing interns' work hours to 60 per week from 80 (now the mandated national maximum). The shorter workweek required a larger staff of interns to spell one another at more frequent intervals. With shorter hours, the interns got more sleep at home, dozed off less at work and made considerably fewer bad mistakes in patient care.

Why should such an obvious finding need an elaborate controlled study to establish? Why should it generate not only two long articles in the world's most prestigious medical journal, but also three long, passionate editorials? Because the issue here is bigger than just scheduling and manpower.

The progressive shortening of residents' work hours spells nothing less than a change in the ethos of medicine itself. It means the end of Dr. Kildare, Superstar— that lone, heroic healer, omniscient, omnipotent and ever-present. It means a revolution in the complex medical hierarchy that sustained him. Willy-nilly, medicine is becoming democratized, a team sport.

We can only hope the revolution will be bloodless. Everything will have to change. Doctors will have to learn to work well with others. They will have to learn to write and speak with enough clarity and precision so that the patient's story remains accurate as care passes from hand to hand. They will have to stop saying "my patient" and begin to say "our patient" instead.

It may be, when the dust settles, that the system will be more functional, less error-prone. It may be that we will simply have substituted one set of problems for another.

We may even find that nothing much has changed. Even in the Harvard data, there was an impressive range in the hours that the interns under study worked. Some logged in over 90 hours in their 80-hour workweek. Some put in 75 instead.

Medicine has always attracted a wide spectrum of individuals, from the lazy and disaffected to the deeply committed. Even draconian scheduling policies may not change basic personality traits, or the kind of doctors that interns grow up to be.

My month with the intern of the past and the intern of the future certainly argues for the power of the individual work ethic. Try as I might, it was not within my power to modify the way either of them functioned. The woman cared too much. The man cared too little. She worked too hard, and he could not be prodded into working hard enough. They both made careless mistakes. When patients died, the man shrugged and the woman cried. If for no other reason than that one, let us hope that the medicine of the future still has room for people like her.

Pure Fancy

People who like this sort of thing
Will find this is the sort of thing they like

Abraham Lincoln

The Masque of the Red Death

Edgar Allen Poe

THE "Red Death" had long devastated the country. No pestilence had ever been so fatal, or so hideous. Blood was its Avatar and its seal — the redness and the horror of blood. There were sharp pains, and sudden dizziness, and then profuse bleeding at the pores, with dissolution. The scarlet stains upon the body and especially upon the face of the victim, were the pest ban which shut him out from the aid and from the sympathy of his fellow-men. And the whole seizure, progress and termination of the disease, were the incidents of half an hour.

But the Prince Prospero was happy and dauntless and sagacious. When his dominions were half depopulated, he summoned to his presence a thousand hale and light-hearted friends from among the knights and dames of his court, and with these retired to the deep seclusion of one of his castellated abbeys. This was an extensive and magnificent structure, the creation of the prince's own eccentric yet august taste. A strong and lofty wall girdled it in. This wall had gates of iron. The courtiers, having entered, brought furnaces and massy hammers and welded the bolts. They resolved to leave means neither of ingress or egress to the sudden impulses of despair or of frenzy from within. The abbey was amply provisioned. With such precautions the courtiers might bid defiance to contagion. The external world could take care of itself. In the meantime it was folly to grieve, or to think. The prince had provided all the appliances of pleasure. There were buffoons, there were improvisatori, there were ballet-dancers, there were musicians, there was Beauty, there was wine. All these and security were within. Without was the "Red Death."

It was toward the close of the fifth or sixth month of his seclusion, and while the pestilence raged most furiously abroad, that the Prince Prospero entertained his thousand friends at a masked ball of the most unusual magnificence.

It was a voluptuous scene, that masquerade. But first let me tell of the rooms in which it was held. There were seven — an imperial suite. In many palaces, however, such suites form a long and straight vista, while the folding doors slide back nearly to the walls on either hand, so that the view of the whole extent is scarcely impeded. Here the case was very different; as might have been expected from the duke's love of the bizarre. The apartments were so irregularly disposed that the vision embraced but little more than one at a time. There was a sharp turn at every twenty or thirty yards, and at each turn a novel effect. To the right and left, in the middle of each wall, a tall and narrow Gothic window looked out upon a closed corridor which pursued the windings of the suite. These windows were of stained glass whose color varied in accordance with the prevailing hue of the decorations of the chamber into which it opened. That at the eastern extremity was hung, for example, in blue — and vividly blue were its windows. The second chamber was purple in its ornaments and tapestries, and here the panes were purple. The third was green throughout, and so were the casements. The fourth was furnished and lighted with orange — the fifth with white — the sixth with violet. The seventh apartment was closely shrouded in black velvet tapestries that hung all over the ceiling and down the walls, falling in heavy folds upon a carpet of the same material and hue. But in this chamber only, the color of the windows failed to correspond with the decorations. The panes here were scarlet — a deep blood color. Now in no one of the seven apartments was there any lamp or candelabrum, amid the profusion of golden ornaments that lay scattered to and fro or depended from the roof. There was no light of any kind emanating from lamp or candle within the suite of chambers. But in the corridors that followed the suite, there stood, opposite to each window, a heavy tripod, bearing a brazier of fire that protected its rays through the tinted glass and so glaringly illumined the room. And thus were produced a multitude of gaudy and fantastic appearances. But in the western or black chamber the effect of the fire-light that streamed upon the dark hangings through the blood-tinted panes, was ghastly in the extreme, and produced so wild a look upon the countenances of those who entered, that there were few of the company bold enough to set foot within its precincts at all.

It was in this apartment, also, that there stood against the western wall, a gigantic clock of ebony. Its pendulum swung to and fro with a dull, heavy, monotonous clang; and when the minute-hand made the circuit of the face, and the hour was to be stricken, there came from the brazen lungs of the clock a sound which was clear and loud and deep and exceedingly musical, but of so peculiar a note and emphasis that, at each lapse of an hour, the musicians of the orchestra were constrained to pause, momentarily, in their performance, to hearken to the sound; and thus the waltzers perforce ceased their evolutions; and there was a brief disconcert of the whole gay company; and, while the chimes of the clock yet rang, it was observed that the giddiest grew pale, and the more aged and sedate passed their hands over their brows as if in confused reverie or meditation. But when the echoes had fully ceased, a light laughter at once pervaded the assembly; the musicians looked at each other and smiled as if at their own nervousness and folly, and made whispering vows, each to the other, that the next chiming of the clock should produce in them no similar emotion; and then, after the lapse of sixty minutes, (which embrace three thousand and six hundred seconds of the Time that flies,) there came yet another chiming of the clock, and then were the same disconcert and tremulousness and meditation as before.

But, in spite of these things, it was a gay and magnificent revel. The tastes of the duke were peculiar. He had a fine eye for colors and effects. He disregarded the decora of mere fashion. His plans were bold and fiery, and his conceptions glowed with barbaric lustre. There are some who would have thought him mad. His followers felt that he was not. It was necessary to hear and see and touch him to be sure that he was not.

He had directed, in great part, the moveable embellishments of the seven chambers, upon occasion of this great fete; and it was his own guiding taste which had given character to the masqueraders. Be sure they were grotesque. There were much glare and glitter and piquancy and phantasm — much of what has been since seen in "Hernani." There were arabesque figures with unsuited limbs and appointments. There were delirious fancies such as the madman fashions. There was much of the beautiful, much of the wanton, much of the bizarre, something of the terrible, and not a little of that which might have excited disgust. To and fro in the seven chambers there stalked, in fact, a multitude of dreams. And these — the dreams — writhed in and about, taking hue from the rooms, and causing the wild music of the orchestra to seem as the echo of their steps. And, anon, there strikes the ebony clock which stands in the hall of the velvet. And then, for a moment, all is still, and all is silent save the voice of the clock. The dreams are stiff-frozen as they stand. But the echoes of the chime die away — they have endured but an instant — and a light, half-subdued laughter floats after them as they depart. And now again the music swells, and the dreams live, and writhe to and fro more merrily than ever, taking hue from the many-tinted windows through which stream the rays from the tripods. But to the chamber which lies most westwardly of the seven, there are now none of the maskers who venture; for the night is waning away; and there flows a ruddier light through the blood-colored panes; and the blackness of the sable drapery appals; and to him whose foot falls upon the sable carpet, there comes from the near clock of ebony a muffled peal more solemnly emphatic than any which reaches their ears who indulge in the more remote gaieties of the other apartments.

But these other apartments were densely crowded, and in them beat feverishly the heart of life. And the revel went whirlingly on, until at length there commenced the sounding of midnight upon the clock. And then the music ceased, as I have told; and the evolutions of the waltzers were quieted; and there was an uneasy cessation of all things as before. But now there were twelve strokes to be sounded by the bell of the clock; and thus it happened, perhaps, that more of thought crept, with more of time, into the meditations of the thoughtful among those who revelled. And thus, too, it happened, perhaps, that before the last echoes of the last chime had utterly sunk into silence, there were many individuals in the crowd who had found leisure to become aware of the presence of a masked figure which had arrested the attention of no single individual before. And the rumor of this new presence having spread itself whisperingly around, there arose at length from the whole company a buzz, or murmur, expressive of disapprobation and surprise — then, finally, of terror, of horror, and of disgust.

In an assembly of phantasms such as I have painted, it may well be supposed that no ordinary appearance could have excited such sensation. In truth the masquerade license of the night was nearly unlimited; but the figure in question had out-Heroded Herod, and gone beyond the bounds of even the prince's indefinite decorum. There are chords in the hearts of the most reckless which cannot be touched without emotion. Even with the utterly lost, to whom life and death are equally jests, there are matters of which no jest can be made. The whole company, indeed, seemed now deeply to feel that in the costume and bearing of the stranger neither wit nor propriety existed. The figure was tall and gaunt, and shrouded from head to foot in the habiliments of the grave. The mask which concealed the visage was made so nearly to resemble the countenance of a stiffened corpse that the closest scrutiny must have had difficulty in detecting the cheat. And yet all this might have been endured, if not approved, by the mad revellers around. But the mummer had gone so far as to assume the type of the Red Death. His vesture was dabbled in blood — and his broad brow, with all the features of the face, was besprinkled with the scarlet horror.

When the eyes of Prince Prospero fell upon this spectral image (which with a slow and solemn movement, as if more fully to sustain its role, stalked to and fro among the waltzers) he was seen to be convulsed, in the first moment with a strong shudder either of terror or distaste; but, in the next, his brow reddened with rage.

"Who dares?" he demanded hoarsely of the courtiers who stood near him — "who dares insult us with this blasphemous mockery? Seize him and unmask him — that we may know whom we have to hang at sunrise, from the battlements!"

It was in the eastern or blue chamber in which stood the Prince Prospero as he uttered these words. They rang throughout the seven rooms loudly and clearly —

for the prince was a bold and robust man, and the music had become hushed at the waving of his hand.

It was in the blue room where stood the prince, with a group of pale courtiers by his side. At first, as he spoke, there was a slight rushing movement of this group in the direction of the intruder, who at the moment was also near at hand, and now, with deliberate and stately step, made closer approach to the speaker. But from a certain nameless awe with which the mad assumptions of the mummer had inspired the whole party, there were found none who put forth hand to seize him; so that, unimpeded, he passed within a yard of the prince's person; and, while the vast assembly, as if with one impulse, shrank from the centres of the rooms to the walls, he made his way uninterruptedly, but with the same solemn and measured step which had distinguished him from the first, through the blue chamber to the purple — through the purple to the green — through the green to the orange — through this again to the white — and even thence to the violet, ere a decided movement had been made to arrest him. It was then, however, that the Prince Prospero, maddening with rage and the shame of his own momentary cowardice, rushed hurriedly through the six chambers, while none followed him on account of a deadly terror that had seized upon all. He bore aloft a drawn dagger, and had approached, in rapid impetuosity, to within three or four feet of the retreating fig-ure, when the latter, having attained the extremity of the velvet apartment, turned suddenly and confronted his pursuer. There was a sharp cry — and the dagger dropped gleaming upon the sable carpet, upon which, instantly afterwards, fell prostrate in death the Prince Prospero. Then, summoning the wild courage of despair, a throng of the revellers at once threw themselves into the black apart-ment, and, seizing the mummer, whose tall figure stood erect and motionless within the shadow of the ebony clock, gasped in unutterable horror at finding the grave-cerements and corpse-like mask which they handled with so violent a rude-ness, untenanted by any tangible form.

And now was acknowledged the presence of the Red Death. He had come like a thief in the night. And one by one dropped the revellers in the blood-bedewed halls of their revel, and died each in the despairing posture of his fall. And the life of the ebony clock went out with that of the last of the gay. And the flames of the tripods expired. And Darkness and Decay and the Red Death held illimitable dominion over all.

Dr. Heidegger's Experiment

Nathaniel Hawthorne

That very singular man, old Dr. Heidegger, once invited four venerable friends to meet him in his study. There were three white-bearded gentlemen, Mr. Medbourne, Colonel Killigrew, and Mr. Gascoigne, and a withered gentlewoman, whose name was the Widow Wycherly. They were all melancholy old creatures, who had been unfortunate in life, and whose greatest misfortune it was that they were not long ago in their graves. Mr. Medbourne, in the vigor of his age, had been a prosperous merchant, but had lost his all by a frantic speculation, and was now little better than a mendicant. Colonel Killigrew had wasted his best years, and his health and substance, in the pursuit of sinful pleasures, which had given birth to a brood of pains, such as the gout, and divers other torments of soul and body. Mr. Gascoigne was a ruined politician, a man of evil fame, or at least had been so till time had buried him from the knowledge of the present generation, and made him obscure instead of infamous. As for the Widow Wycherly, tradition tells us that she was a great beauty in her day; but, for a long while past, she had lived in deep seclusion, on account of certain scandalous stories which had prejudiced the gentry of the town against her. It is a circumstance worth mentioning that each of these three old gentlemen, Mr. Medbourne, Colonel Killigrew, and Mr. Gascoigne, were early lovers of the Widow Wycherly, and had once been on the point of cutting each other's throats for her sake. And, before proceeding further, I will merely hint that Dr. Heidegger and all his foul guests were sometimes thought to be a little beside themselves, — as is not unfrequently the case with old people, when worried either by present troubles or woful recollections.

"My dear old friends," said Dr. Heidegger, motioning them to be seated, "I am desirous of your assistance in one of those little experiments with which I amuse myself here in my study."

If all stories were true, Dr. Heidegger's study must have been a very curious place. It was a dim, old-fashioned chamber, festooned with cobwebs, and besprinkled with antique dust. Around the walls stood several oaken bookcases, the lower shelves of which were filled with rows of gigantic folios and black-letter quartos, and the upper with little parchment-covered duodecimos. Over the central book-case was a bronze bust of Hippocrates, with which, according to some authorities, Dr. Heidegger was accustomed to hold consultations in all difficult cases of his practice. In the obscurest corner of the room stood a tall and narrow oaken closet, with its door ajar, within which doubtfully appeared a skeleton. Between two of the bookcases hung a looking-glass, presenting its high and dusty plate within a tarnished gilt frame. Among many wonderful stories related of this mirror, it was fabled that the spirits of all the doctor's deceased patients dwelt within its verge, and would stare him in the face whenever he looked thitherward. The opposite side of the chamber was ornamented with the full-length portrait of a young lady, arrayed in the faded magnificence of silk, satin, and brocade, and with a visage as faded as her dress. Above half a century ago, Dr. Heidegger had been on the point of marriage with this young lady; but, being affected with some slight disorder, she had swallowed one of her lover's prescriptions, and died on the bridal evening. The greatest curiosity of the study remains to be mentioned; it was a ponderous folio volume, bound in black leather, with massive silver clasps. There were no letters on the back, and nobody could tell the title of the book. But it was well known to be a book of magic; and once, when a chambermaid had lifted it, merely to brush away the dust, the skeleton had rattled in its closet, the picture of the young lady had stepped one foot upon the floor, and several ghastly faces had peeped forth from the mirror; while the brazen head of Hippocrates frowned, and said, — "Forbear!"

Such was Dr. Heidegger's study. On the summer afternoon of our tale a small round table, as black as ebony, stood in the centre of the room, sustaining a cut-glass vase of beautiful form and elaborate workmanship. The sunshine came through the window, between the heavy festoons of two faded damask curtains, and fell directly across this vase; so that a mild splendor was reflected from it on the ashen visages of the five old people who sat around. Four champagne glasses were also on the table.

"My dear old friends," repeated Dr. Heidegger, "may I reckon on your aid in performing an exceedingly curious experiment?"

Now Dr. Heidegger was a very strange old gentleman, whose eccentricity had become the nucleus for a thousand fantastic stories. Some of these fables, to my shame be it spoken, might possibly be traced back to my own veracious self; and if any passages of the present tale should startle the reader's faith, I must be content to bear the stigma of a fiction monger.

When the doctor's four guests heard him talk of his proposed experiment, they anticipated nothing more wonderful than the murder of a mouse in an air pump, or the examination of a cobweb by the microscope, or some similar nonsense, with which he was constantly in the habit of pestering his intimates. But without waiting for a reply, Dr. Heidegger hobbled across the chamber, and returned with the same ponderous folio, bound in black leather, which common report affirmed to be a book of magic. Undoing the silver clasps, he opened the volume, and took from among its black-letter pages a rose, or what was once a rose, though now the green leaves and crimson petals had assumed one brownish hue, and the ancient flower seemed ready to crumble to dust in the doctor's hands.

"This rose," said Dr. Heidegger, with a sigh, "this same withered and crumbling flower, blossomed five and fifty years ago. It was given me by Sylvia Ward, whose portrait hangs yonder; and I meant to wear it in my bosom at our wedding. Five and fifty years it has been treasured between the leaves of this old volume. Now, would you deem it possible that this rose of half a century could ever bloom again?"

"Nonsense!" said the Widow Wycherly, with a peevish toss of her head. "You might as well ask whether an old woman's wrinkled face could ever bloom again."

"See!" answered Dr. Heidegger.

He uncovered the vase, and threw the faded rose into the water which it contained. At first, it lay lightly on the surface of the fluid, appearing to imbibe none of its moisture. Soon, however, a singular change began to be visible. The crushed and dried petals stirred, and assumed a deepening tinge of crimson, as if the flower were reviving from a deathlike slumber; the slender stalk and twigs of foliage became green; and there was the rose of half a century, looking as fresh as when Sylvia Ward had first given it to her lover. It was scarcely full blown; for some of its delicate red leaves curled modestly around its moist bosom, within which two or three dewdrops were sparkling.

"That is certainly a very pretty deception," said the doctor's friends; carelessly, however, for they had witnessed greater miracles at a conjurer's show; "pray how was it effected?"

"Did you never hear of the 'Fountain of Youth?" asked Dr. Heidegger, "which Ponce De Leon, the Spanish adventurer, went in search of two or three centuries ago?"

"But did Ponce De Leon ever find it?" said the Widow Wycherly.

"No," answered Dr. Heidegger, "for he never sought it in the right place. The famous Fountain of Youth, if I am rightly informed, is situated in the southern part of the Floridian peninsula, not far from Lake Macaco. Its source is overshadowed by several gigantic magnolias, which, though numberless centuries old, have been kept as fresh as violets by the virtues of this wonderful water. An acquaintance of mine, knowing my curiosity in such matters, has sent me what you see in the vase."

"Ahem!" said Colonel Killigrew, who believed not a word of the doctor's story; "and what may be the effect of this fluid on the human frame?"

"You shall judge for yourself, my dear colonel," replied Dr. Heidegger; "and all of you, my respected friends, are welcome to so much of this admirable fluid as may restore to you the bloom of youth. For my own part, having had much trouble in growing old, I am in no hurry to grow young again. With your permission, therefore, I will merely watch the progress of the experiment."

While he spoke, Dr. Heidegger had been filling the four champagne glasses with the water of the Fountain of Youth. It was apparently impregnated with an effervescent gas, for little bubbles were continually ascending from the depths of the glasses, and bursting in silvery spray at the surface. As the liquor diffused a pleasant perfume, the old people doubted not that it possessed cordial and comfortable properties; and though utter sceptics as to its rejuvenescent power, they were inclined to swallow it at once. But Dr. Heidegger besought them to stay a moment.

"Before you drink, my respectable old friends," said he, "it would be well that, with the experience of a lifetime to direct you, you should draw up a few general rules for your guidance, in passing a second time through the perils of youth. Think what a sin and shame it would be, if, with your peculiar advantages, you should not become patterns of virtue and wisdom to all the young people of the age!"

The doctor's four venerable friends made him no answer, except by a feeble and tremulous laugh; so very ridiculous was the idea that, knowing how closely repentance treads behind the steps of error, they should ever go astray again.

"Drink, then," said the doctor, bowing: "I rejoice that I have so well selected the subjects of my experiment."

With palsied hands, they raised the glasses to their lips. The liquor, if it really possessed such virtues as Dr. Heidegger imputed to it, could not have been bestowed on four human beings who needed it more wofully. They looked as if they had never known what youth or pleasure was, but had been the offspring of Nature's dotage, and always the gray, decrepit, sapless, miserable creatures, who now sat stooping round the doctor's table, without life enough in their souls or bodies to be animated even by the prospect of growing young again. They drank off the water, and replaced their glasses on the table.

Assuredly there was an almost immediate improvement in the aspect of the party, not unlike what might have been produced by a glass of generous wine, together with a sudden glow of cheerful sunshine brightening over all their visages at once. There was a healthful suffusion on their cheeks, instead of the ashen hue that had made them look so corpse-like. They gazed at one another, and fancied that some magic power had really begun to smooth away the deep and sad inscriptions which Father Time had been so long engraving on their brows. The Widow Wycherly adjusted her cap, for she felt almost like a woman again.

"Give us more of this wondrous water!" cried they, eagerly. "We are younger — but we are still too old! Quick — give us more!"

"Patience, patience!" quoth Dr. Heidegger, who sat watching the experiment with philosophic coolness. "You have been a long time growing old. Surely, you might be content to grow young in half an hour! But the water is at your service."

Again he filled their glasses with the liquor of youth, enough of which still remained in the vase to turn half the old people in the city to the age of their own grandchildren. While the bubbles were yet sparkling on the brim, the doctor's four guests snatched their glasses from the table, and swallowed the contents at a single gulp. Was it delusion? even while the draught was passing down their throats, it seemed to have wrought a change on their whole systems. Their eyes grew clear and bright; a dark shade deepened among their silvery locks, they sat around the table, three gentlemen of middle age, and a woman, hardly beyond her buxom prime.

"My dear widow, you are charming!" cried Colonel Killigrew, whose eyes had been fixed upon her face, while the shadows of age were flitting from it like darkness from the crimson daybreak.

The fair widow knew, of old, that Colonel Killigrew's compliments were not always measured by sober truth; so she started up and ran to the mirror, still dreading that the ugly visage of an old woman would meet her gaze. Meanwhile, the three gentlemen behaved in such a manner as proved that the water of the Fountain of Youth possessed some intoxicating qualities; unless, indeed, their exhilaration of spirits were merely a lightsome dizziness caused by the sudden removal of the weight of years. Mr. Gascoigne's mind seemed to run on political topics, but whether relating to the past, present, or future, could not easily be determined, since the same ideas and phrases have been in vogue these fifty years. Now he rattled forth full-throated sentences about patriotism, national glory, and the people's right; now he muttered some perilous stuff or other, in a sly and doubtful whisper, so cautiously that even his own conscience could scarcely catch the secret; and now, again, he spoke in measured accents, and a deeply deferential tone, as if a royal ear were listening to his well-turned periods. Colonel Killigrew all this time had been trolling forth a jolly bottle song, and ringing his glass in symphony with the chorus, while his eyes wandered toward the buxom figure of the Widow Wycherly. On the other side of the table, Mr. Medbourne was involved in a calculation of dollars and cents, with which was strangely intermingled a project for supplying the East Indies with ice, by harnessing a team of whales to the polar icebergs.

As for the Widow Wycherly, she stood before the mirror courtesying and simpering to her own image, and greeting it as the friend whom she loved better than all the world beside. She thrust her face close to the glass, to see whether some long-remembered wrinkle or crow's foot had indeed vanished. She examined whether the snow had so entirely melted from her hair that the venerable cap could be safely thrown aside. At last, turning briskly away, she came with a sort of dancing step to the table.

"My dear old doctor," cried she, "pray favor me with another glass!"

"Certainly, my dear madam, certainly!" replied the complaisant doctor; "see! I have already filled the glasses."

There, in fact, stood the four glasses, brimful of this wonderful water, the delicate spray of which, as it effervesced from the surface, resembled the tremulous glitter of diamonds. It was now so nearly sunset that the chamber had grown duskier than ever; but a mild and moonlike splendor gleamed from within the vase, and rested alike on the four guests and on the doctor's venerable figure. He sat in a high-backed, elaborately-carved, oaken arm-chair, with a gray dignity of aspect that might have well befitted that very Father Time, whose power had never been disputed, save by this fortunate company. Even while quaffing the third draught of the Fountain of Youth, they were almost awed by the expression of his mysterious visage.

But, the next moment, the exhilarating gush of young life shot through their veins. They were now in the happy prime of youth. Age, with its miserable train of cares and sorrows and diseases, was remembered only as the trouble of a dream, from which they had joyously awoke. The fresh gloss of the soul, so early lost, and without which the world's successive scenes had been but a gallery of faded pictures, again threw its enchantment over all their prospects. They felt like new-created beings in a new-created universe.

"We are young! We are young!" they cried exultingly.

Youth, like the extremity of age, had effaced the strongly-marked characteristics of middle life, and mutually assimilated them all. They were a group of merry youngsters, almost maddened with the exuberant frolicsomeness of their years. The most singular effect of their gayety was an impulse to mock the infirmity and decrepitude of which they had so lately been the victims. They laughed loudly at their old-fashioned attire, the wide-skirted coats and flapped waistcoats of the young men, and the ancient cap and gown of the blooming girl. One limped across the floor like a gouty grandfather; one set a pair of spectacles astride of his nose, and pretended to pore over the black-letter pages of the book of magic; a third seated himself in an arm-chair, and strove to imitate the venerable dignity of Dr. Heidegger. Then all shouted mirthfully, and leaped about the room. The Widow Wycherly — if so fresh a damsel could be called a widow-tripped up to the doctor's chair, with a mischievous merriment in her rosy face.

"Doctor, you dear old soul," cried she, "get up and dance with me!" And then the four young people laughed louder than ever, to think what a queer figure the poor old doctor would cut.

"Pray excuse me," answered the doctor quietly. "I am old and rheumatic, and my dancing days were over long ago. But either of these gay young gentlemen will be glad of so pretty a partner."

"Dance with me, Clara!" cried Colonel Killigrew.

"No, no, I will be her partner!" shouted Mr. Gascoigne.

"She promised me her hand, fifty years ago!" exclaimed Mr. Medbourne.

They all gathered round her. One caught both her hands in his passionate grasp another threw his arm about her waist — the third buried his hand among the glossy curls that clustered beneath the widow's cap. Blushing, panting, struggling, chiding, laughing, her warm breath fanning each of their faces by turns, she strove to disengage herself, yet still remained in their triple embrace. Never was there a livelier picture of youthful rivalship, with bewitching beauty for the prize. Yet, by a strange deception, owing to the duskiness of the chamber, and the antique dresses which they still wore, the tall mirror is said to have reflected the figures of the three old, gray, withered grandsires, ridiculously contending for the skinny ugli-ness of a shrivelled grandam.

But they were young: their burning passions proved them so. Inflamed to madness by the coquetry of the girl-widow, who neither granted nor quite withheld her favors, the three rivals began to interchange threatening glances. Still keeping hold of the fair prize, they grappled fiercely at one another's throats. As they struggled to and fro, the table was over-turned, and the vase dashed into a thousand fragments. The precious Water of Youth flowed in a bright stream across the floor, moistening the wings of a butterfly, which, grown old in the decline of summer, had alighted there to die. The insect fluttered lightly through the chamber, and settled on the snowy head of Dr. Heidegger.

"Come, come, gentlemen! — come, Madam Wycherly," exclaimed the doctor, "I really must protest against this riot."

They stood still and shivered; for it seemed as if gray Time were calling them back from their sunny youth, far down into the chill and darksome vale of years. They looked at old Dr. Heidegger, who sat in his carved arm-chair, holding the rose of half a century, which he had rescued from among the fragments of the shattered vase. At the motion of his hand, the four rioters resumed their seats; the more readily, because their violent exertions had wearied them, youthful though they were.

"My poor Sylvia's rose!" ejaculated Dr. Heidegger, holding it in the light of the sunset clouds; "it appears to be fading again."

And so it was. Even while the party were looking at it, the flower continued to shrivel up, till it became as dry and fragile as when the doctor had first thrown it into the vase. He shook off the few drops of moisture which clung to its petals.

"I love it as well thus as in its dewy freshness," observed he, pressing the withered rose to his withered lips. While he spoke, the butterfly fluttered down from the doctor's snowy head, and fell upon the floor.

His guests shivered again. A strange chillness, whether of the body or spirit they could not tell, was creeping gradually over them all. They gazed at one another, and fancied that each fleeting moment snatched away a charm, and left a deepening furrow where none had been before. Was it an illusion? Had the changes of a lifetime been crowded into so brief a space, and were they now four aged people, sitting with their old friend, Dr. Heidegger?

"Are we grown old again, so soon?" cried they, dolefully.

In truth they had. The Water of Youth possessed merely a virtue more transient than that of wine. The delirium which it created had effervesced away. Yes! they were old again. With a shuddering impulse, that showed her a woman still, the widow clasped her skinny hands before her face, and wished that the coffin lid were over it, since it could be no longer beautiful.

"Yes, friends, ye are old again," said Dr. Heidegger, "and lo! the Water of Youth is all lavished on the ground. Well — I bemoan it not; for if the fountain gushed at my very doorstep, I would not stoop to bathe my lips in it — no, though its delirium were for years instead of moments. Such is the lesson ye have taught me!"

But the doctor's four friends had taught no such lesson to themselves. They resolved forthwith to make a pilgrimage to Florida, and quaff at morning, noon, and night, from the Fountain of Youth.

The Ones Who Walk Away from Omelas

Ursula Le Guin

With a clamor of bells that set the swallows soaring, the Festival of Summer came to the city Omelas, bright-towered by the sea. The rigging of the boats in harbor sparkled with flags. In the streets between houses with red roofs and painted walls, between old moss-grown gardens and under avenues of trees, past great parks and public buildings, processions moved. Some were decorous: old people in long stiff robes of mauve and grey, grave master workmen, quiet, merry women carrying their babies and chatting as they walked. In other streets the music beat faster, a shimmering of gong and tambourine, and the people went dancing, the procession was a dance. Children dodged in and out, their high calls rising like the swallows' crossing flights over the music and thc singing. All the processions wound towards the north side of the city, where on the great water-meadow called the Green Fields boys and girls, naked in the bright air, with mud-stained feet and ankles and long, lithe arms, exercised their restive horses before the race. The horses wore no gear at all but a halter without bit. Their manes were braided with streamers of silver, gold, and green. They flared their nostrils and pranced and boasted to one another; they were vastly excited, the horse being the only animal who has adopted our ceremonies as his own. Far off to the north and west the mountains stood up half encircling Omelas on her bay. The air of morning was so clear that the snow still crowning the Eighteen Peaks burned with white-gold fire across the miles of sunlit air, under the dark blue of the sky. There was just enough wind to make the banners that marked the racecourse snap and flutter now and then. In the silence of the broad green meadows one could hear the music winding through the city streets, farther and nearer and ever approaching, a cheerful faint sweetness of the air that from time to time trembled and gathered together and broke out into the great joyous clanging of the bells.

Joyous! How is one to tell about joy? How describe the citizens of Omelas?

They were not simple folk, you see, though they were happy. But we do not say the words of cheer much any more. All smiles have become archaic. Given a description such as this one tends to make certain assumptions. Given a description such as this one tends to look next for the King, mounted on a splendid stallion and surrounded by his noble knights, or perhaps in a golden litter borne by great-muscled slaves. But there was no king. They did not use swords, or keep slaves. They were not barbarians. I do not know the rules and laws of their society, but I suspect that they were singularly few. As they did without monarchy and slavery, so they also got on without the stock exchange, the advertisement, the secret police, and the bomb. Yet I repeat that these were not simple folk, not dulcet shepherds, noble savages, bland utopians. They were not less complex than us. The trouble is that we have a bad habit, encouraged by pedants and sophisticates, of considering happiness as something rather stupid. Only pain is intellectual, only evil interesting. This is the treason of the artist: a refusal to admit the banality of evil and the terrible boredom of pain. If you can't lick 'em, join 'em. If it hurts, repeat it. But to praise despair is to condemn delight, to embrace violence is to lose hold of everything else. We have almost lost hold, we can no longer describe a happy man, nor make any celebration of joy. How can I tell you about the people of Omelas? They were not naïve and happy children—though their children were, in fact, happy. They were mature, intelligent, passionate adults whose lives were not wretched. O miracle! but I wish I could describe it better. I wish I could convince you. Omelas sounds in my words like a city in a fairy tale, long ago and far away, once upon a time. Perhaps it would be best if you imagined it as your own fancy bids, assuming it will rise to the occasion, for certainly I cannot suit you all. For instance, how about technology? I think that there would be no cars or helicopters in and above the streets; this follows from the fact that the people of Omelas are happy people. Happiness is based on a just discrimination of what is necessary, what is neither necessary nor destructive, and what is destructive. In the middle category, however—that of the unnecessary but undestructive, that of comfort, luxury, exuberance, etc.—they could perfectly well have central heating, subway trains, washing machines, and all kinds of marvelous devices not yet invented here, floating light-sources, fuelless power, a cure for the common cold. Or they could have none of that: it doesn't matter. As you like it. I incline to think that people from towns up and down the coast have been coming in to Omelas during the last days before the Festival on very fast little trains and double-decked trams, and that the train station of Omelas is actually the handsomest building in town, though plainer than the magnificent Farmers' Market. But even granted trains, I fear the Omelas so far strikes some of you as goody-goody. Smiles, bells, parades, horses, bleh. If so, please add an orgy. If an orgy would help, don't hesitate. Let us not, however, have temples from which issue beautiful nude priests and priestesses already half in ecstasy and ready to copulate with any man or woman, lover or stranger, who desires union with the deep godhead of the blood, although that was my first idea. But really it would be better not to have any temples in Omelas—at least, not manned temples. Religion yes, clergy no. Surely the beautiful nudes can just wander about, offering themselves like divine soufflés to the hunger of the needy and the rapture of the flesh. Let them join the processions. Let tambourines be struck above the copulations, and the glory of desire be proclaimed upon the gongs, and (a not unimportant point) let the offspring of these delightful rituals be beloved and looked after by all. One thing I know there is none of in Omelas is guilt. But what else should there be? I thought at first there were no drugs, but that is puritanical. For those who like it, the faint insistent sweetness of drooz may perfume the ways of the city, drooz which first brings a great lightness and brilliance to the mind and limbs, and then after some hours a dreamy languor, and wonderful visions at last of the very arcana and inmost secrets of the Universe, as well as exciting the pleasure of sex beyond all belief; and it is not habit-forming. For more modest tastes I think there ought to be beer. What else, what else belongs in the joyous city? The sense of victory, surely, the celebration of courage. But as we did without clergy, let us do without soldiers. The joy built upon successful slaughter is not the right kind of joy; it will not do; it is fearful and it is trivial. A boundless and generous contentment, a magnanimous triumph felt not against some outer enemy but in communion with the finest and fairest in the souls of all men everywhere and the splendor of the world's summer: this is what swells the hearts of the people of Omelas, and the victory they celebrate is that of life. I really don't think many of them need to take drooz.

Most of the processions have reached the Green Fields by now. A marvelous smell of cooking goes forth from the red and blue tents of the provisioners. The faces of small children are amiably sticky; in the benign grey beard of a man a couple of crumbs of rich pastry are entangled. The youths and girls have mounted their horses and are beginning to group around the starting line of the course. An old woman, small, fat, and laughing, is passing out flowers from a basket, and tall young men wear her flowers in their shining hair. A child of nine or ten sits at the edge of the crowd, alone, playing on a wooden flute. People pause to listen, and they smile, but they do not speak to him, for he never ceases playing and never sees them, his dark eyes wholly rapt in the sweet, thin magic of the tune.

He finishes, and slowly lowers his hands holding the wooden flute.

As if that little private silence were the signal, all at once a trumpet sounds from the pavilion near the starting line: imperious, melancholy, piercing. The horses rear on their slender legs, and some of them neigh in answer. Sober-faced, the young riders stroke the horses' necks and soothe them, whispering, "Quiet, quiet, there my beauty, my hope...." They begin to form in rank along the starting line. The crowds along the racecourse are like a field of grass and flowers in the wind. The Festival of Summer has begun.

Do you believe? Do you accept the festival, the city, the joy? No? Then let me describe one more thing.

In a basement under one of the beautiful public buildings of Omelas, or perhaps in the cellar of one of its spacious private homes, there is a room. It has one locked door, and no window. A little light seeps in dustily between cracks in the boards, secondhand from a cobwebbed window somewhere across the cellar. In one corner of the little room a couple of mops, with stiff, clotted, foul-smelling heads, stand near a rusty bucket. The floor is dirt, a little damp to the touch, as cellar dirt usually is. The room is about three paces long and two wide: a mere broom closet or disused tool room. In the room a child is sitting. It could be a boy or a girl. It looks about six, but actually is nearly ten. It is feeble-minded. Perhaps it was born defective, or perhaps it has become imbecile through fear, malnutrition, and neglect. It picks its nose and occasionally fumbles vaguely with its toes or genitals, as it sits hunched in the corner farthest from the bucket and the two mops. It is afraid of the mops. It finds them horrible. It shuts its eyes, but it knows the mops are still standing there; and the door is locked; and nobody will come. The door is always locked; and nobody ever comes, except that sometimes—the child has no understanding of time or interval—sometimes the door rattles terribly and opens, and a person, or several people, are there. One of them may come in and kick the child to make it stand up. The others never come close, but peer in at it with frightened, disgusted eyes. The food bowl and the water jug are hastily filled, the door is locked, the eyes disappear. The people at the door never say anything, but the child, who has not always lived in the tool room, and can remember sunlight and its mother's voice, sometimes speaks. "I will be good," it says. "Please let me out. I will be good!" They never answer. The child used to scream for help at night, and cry a good deal, but now it only makes a kind of whining, "eh-haa, eh-haa," and it speaks less and less often. It is so thin there are no calves to its legs; its belly protrudes; it lives on a half-bowl of corn meal and grease a day. It is naked. Its buttocks and thighs are a mass of festered sores, as it sits in its own excrement continually.

They all know it is there, all the people of Omelas. Some of them have come to see it, others are content merely to know it is there. They all know that it has to be there. Some of them understand why, and some do not, but they all understand that their happiness, the beauty of their city, the tenderness of their friendships, the health of their children, the wisdom of their scholars, the skill of their makers, even the abundance of their harvest and the kindly weathers of their skies, depend wholly on this child's abominable misery.

This is usually explained to children when they are between eight and twelve, whenever they seem capable of understanding; and most of those who come to see the child are young people, though often enough an adult comes, or comes back, to see the child. No matter how well the matter has been explained to them, these young spectators are always shocked and sickened at the sight. They feel disgust, which they had thought themselves superior to. They feel anger, outrage, impotence, despite all the explanations. They would like to do something for the child. But there is nothing they can do. If the child were brought up into the sunlight out of the vile place, if it were cleaned and fed and comforted, that would be a good thing, indeed; but if it were done, in that day and hour all the prosperity and beauty and delight of Omelas would wither and be destroyed. Those are the terms. To exchange all the goodness and grace of every life in Omelas for that single, small improvement: to throw away the happiness of thousands for the chance of the happiness of one: that would be to let guilt within the walls indeed.

The terms are strict and absolute; there may not even be a kind word spoken to the child.

Often the young people go home in tears, or in a tearless rage, when they have seen the child and faced this terrible paradox. They may brood over it for weeks or years. But as time goes on they begin to realize that even if the child could be released, it would not get much good of its freedom: a little vague pleasure of warmth and food, no doubt, but little more. It is too degraded and imbecile to know any real joy. It has been afraid too long ever to be free of fear. Its habits are too uncouth for it to respond to humane treatment. Indeed, after so long it would probably be wretched without walls about it to protect it, and darkness for its eyes, and its own excrement to sit in. Their tears at the bitter injustice dry when they begin to perceive the terrible justice of reality, and to accept it. Yet it is their tears and anger, the trying of their generosity and the acceptance of their helplessness, which are perhaps the true source of the splendor of their lives. Theirs is no vapid, irresponsible happiness. They know that they, like the child, are not free. They know compassion. It is the existence of the child, and their knowledge of its existence, that makes possible the nobility of their architecture, the poignancy of their music, the profundity of their science. It is because of the child that they are so gentle with children. They know that if the wretched one were not there snivelling in the dark, the other one, the flute-player, could make no joyful music as the young riders line up in their beauty for the race in the sunlight of the first morning of summer.

Now do you believe in them? Are they not more credible? But there is one more thing to tell, and this is quite incredible.

At times one of the adolescent girls or boys who go to see the child does not go home to weep or rage, does not, in fact, go home at all. Sometimes also a man or woman much older falls silent for a day or two, and then leaves home. These people go out into the street, and walk down the street alone. They keep walking, and walk straight out of the city of Omelas, through the beautiful gates. They keep walking across the farmlands of Omelas. Each one goes alone, youth or girl, man or woman. Night falls; the traveler must pass down village streets, between houses with yellow-lit windows, and on out into the darkness of the fields. Each alone, they go west or north, towards the mountains. They go on. They leave Omelas, they walk ahead into the darkness, and they do not come back. The place they go towards is a place even less imaginable to most of us than the city of happiness. I cannot describe it at all. It is possible that it does not exist. But they seem to know where they are going, the ones who walk away from Omelas.

Biographical Sketches and Suggested Further Readings

Bauby, Jean-Dominique (1952–1997) suffered a stroke at the age of 43, which left him with Locked-in Syndrome. He composed and dictated his book the following summer and died ten days after its publication.

Carver, Raymond (1938–1988) revitalized the short story in the 1980's. His style is reminiscent of Kafka, Chekhov, and Hemingway and his first collection, published in 1967, was shortlisted for the National Book Award. His best volume of stories is considered to be *Cathedral*, Vintage Books, 1984.

Chekhov, Anton (1860–1904) a physician, is certainly Russia's greatest short-story writer and has been described by Raymond Carver as "the greatest short story writer who ever lived." A good place to begin: *Chekhov's Doctors: A Collection of Chekhov's Medical Tales*, edited by Jack Coulehan.

Curie, Marie (1867–1934) is the only person to have won two Nobel Prizes in different sciences. She was the first female professor at the University of Paris. Her husband Pierre was killed in a street accident in 1906.

Cushing, Harvey (1869–1939), one of the greatest neurosurgeons of the 20th century, wrote the definitive biography of Osler, which won him the Pulitzer Prize in 1926. Educated at Harvard Medical School and professor of surgery there, his library is at Yale, which is a story in itself.

Featherstone, J.P. (1913–1996) a country doctor, is beloved by Virginian physicians as one of their own. As the story implies, he deeply loved good port, fine cigars, the practice of medicine, and his wife Mary.

Gordon, Mary (1949–) is from New York and attended Barnard College. Her first collection of stories, *Temporary Shelter*, and her three novellas contained in *The Rest of Life*, comprise writing that is very, very fine.

Gramaglia, Tony wrote *From A Burning House: The Aids Project Los Angeles Writers Workshop Collection.* Published in 1996, the book remains in print.

Hawthorne, Nathaniel (1804–1864) graduated from Bowdoin College in Maine where he was a classmate of Longfellow. His best-known novel is *The Scarlet Letter.*

Hemingway, Ernest (1899–1961) received the Pulitzer Prize for *The Old Man and the Sea* and won the Nobel Prize in Literature in 1954. His father was a country doctor in Illinois.

Henook-Makhewe-Kelenaka (1871–1919) was born in a wigwam in Nebraska on the Winnebago reservation. Her name translates into the English "angel" and she is also known by her English name, Angel DeCora. This story, *The Sick Child*, was published in Harper's Magazine in 1899. She became better known as an artist and taught Native American Art at the Carlisle Indian School.

Hippocrates (ca. 460 BC– ca. 370 BC), the father of medicine, was said by ancient Arabic historians to have had a daughter whose skills in medicine rivaled her father's and whose name translated from the Arabic was *Asclepius-like Woman Physician.*

Hugo, Victor (1802–1885) is one of France's great national heroes and arguably one of the greatest novelists of all time. His *Les Miserables* is a must read. On the occasion of his 79th birthday, one of the largest parades in French history was held; the parade took six hours to pass by Hugo, observing from the window of his house in Paris.

Jefferson, Thomas (1743–1826), third president of the United States, a true polymath, wrote the Declaration of Independence, the finest writing one could find anywhere. When President John F. Kennedy welcomed forty-nine Nobel Prize winners to the White House in 1962 he said, "I think this is the most extraordinary collection of talent and of human knowledge that has ever been gathered together at the White House — with the possible exception of when Thomas Jefferson dined alone."

LeGuin, Ursula (1929–) was born in Berkeley and educated at Radcliffe and Columbia. She has honorary degrees from nine universities and is considered one of the greatest writers of science fiction, ever. She has received several Hugo and Nebula Awards and in 2000 was given the Library of Congress Living Legends Award. It is the hope of the editors that this story of hers will haunt caring physicians everywhere.

Lessing, Doris (1919–) was born in Persia and in 2007 became the oldest person ever to win the Nobel Prize in Literature. Her *Prisons We Choose to Live Inside* at 96 pages, is a gem and a must-have, must-read and is still in print. (Jonathan Cape, 1987)

Lewis, Sinclair (1885–1951) was the first American to win the Nobel Prize in Literature, in 1930. His father was a physician in Minnesota. *Arrowsmith* (1925) is a classic, and not just for physicians, and *Babbitt* (1922) was especially praised by the Swedish Academy.

Lincoln, Abraham (1809–1865) was the 16th president of the United States. He was assasinated on April 15, 1865. His most famous speech, The Gettysburg Address, was delivered on November 19, 1863.

Luther Standing Bear (1868–1939), a Lakota Sioux, was born on the Pine Ridge Reservation in South Dakota. He was a hereditary chief of the Dakotas and one of the first students to attend the Carlisle Indian School in Pennsylvania. *My Indian Boyhood*, published by the University of Nebraska Press, is worth finding.

Mates, Susan Onthank won the 1994 John Simmons Short Fiction Award for her short story collection, *The Good Doctor*, from which this piece comes. She is a practicing physician.

Moore, Lorrie is from Glens Fall, NY and graduated from St. Lawrence University. This piece is loosely based on events from her own life. In 2004 she won the Rea Award for the Short Story. She is an English professor at the University of Wisconsin.

More, Thomas (1478–1535), whom G.K. Chesterton called the greatest historical character in English history, was England's 'man for all seasons.' One of the greatest scholars in history, he was beheaded in the Tower of London upon the order of Henry VIII on July 6, 1535. Yes, see the movie with Paul Scofield (1966).

Munthe, Axel (1857–1949), a Swedish physician, studied medicine at the Sorbonne under Charcot. When he went to Naples to help out with the cholera epidemic there, he found and became obsessed with restoring an old villa once owned by the Emperor Tiberius on the island of Capri. It is arguably the most beautiful spot in the world. Read the book, published in 1929 and still in print.

Neruda, Pablo (1904–1973) won the Nobel Prize for Literature in 1971. Chilean, he is considered one of the 20th century's greatest poets. Allende invited him to read his poetry upon his return to Chile after his Nobel Prize acceptance, which he did before 70,000 people. *Il Postino* (1995), a movie based on Neruda's exile, is wonderful.

O'Connor, Frank (1903–1966), arguably Ireland's best short story writer, has been described as that country's most complete man of letters. *A Great Man* is from his *Collected Stories* (Vintage, 1982), a treasure to read.

Osler, William (1849–1919) born in Ontario, received his M.D. from McGill where he became professor before moving on to Penn, then Hopkins, and ultimately to Oxford. Eminently quotable, Osler as a true Renaissance man is captured well in *The Quotable Osler*, ACP Press, 2007.

Pamuk, Orhan (1952–), born in Istanbul, is a Nobel Prize-winning Turkish novelist. His piece contained in this anthology was sent to us by a Turkish physician, Cem Sungur. Awarded the Prize in 2006, he became the first Turkish person to receive any Nobel Prize. He has been a visiting scholar at Columbia and at the University of Iowa and is currently writer in residence at Bard.

Plato (424 BC–348 BC) taught Aristotle and was himself a student of Socrates. 'Plato' is actually a nickname, meaning 'hefty' in Greek, given to him by a wrestling coach. For readability, start with his *Phaedrus*. H.N. Fowler is a good translation.

Poe, Edgar Allen (1809–1849) wrote some great, entertaining short stories, familiar to us all. (Or should be.) Preoccupied with being buried alive, he died a premature death at the age of forty and is buried in Baltimore. Every January 19th, on the anniversary of Poe's birth, for decades someone has left a single rose and a half-consumed bottle of cognac. That person's identity remains unknown.

Price, Reynolds is the James B. Duke Professor of English at Duke University. The author of twenty-five books, his *Collected Stories* is well worth finding. An astrocytoma of the spinal cord left him paraplegic in 1984.

Rice, Grantland (1880–1954) was an early 20th century sports writer.

Rush, Benjamin (1745–1813), a signer of the Declaration of Independence, was professor of medicine at the University of Pennsylvania. He published the first American textbook of chemistry and is credited with the invention of the idea of addiction.

Sacks, Oliver (1933–) was born in London and received his M.D. from Oxford. His father was a general practitioner and his mother, a surgeon. A renowned author, Sacks is professor of neurology at Columbia.

Selzer, Richard was born and raised in Troy, NY where his father was a general practitioner. He retired as professor of surgery from Yale in 1985 and his book, *Letters to a Young Doctor*, from which *Brute* comes, is one of his best books.

Solzhenitsyn, Alexandr (1918–), Russian novelist, won the Nobel Prize in Literature in 1970. He began writing during his imprisonment in a Soviet labor camp beginning in 1945, and his experiences there, contained in *The First Circle*, were published in the West in 1968. His own experience with stomach cancer formed the basis for his novel *Cancer Ward*, from which this excerpt comes.

Thomas, Lewis (1913–1993) won the National Book Award in 1974 for his first collection of essays, *The Lives of a Cell: Notes of a Biology Watcher*. He served as Dean of Yale and NYU, as well as President of Memorial Sloan-Kettering Institute.

Twain, Mark (1835–1910), described by Faulkner as the father of American literature, is well known to all American readers and his popularity has never diminished. A physician who felt it should be read by all physicians sent in this excerpt from *Life On The Mississippi*.

Verghese, Abraham (1955–), the author of *My Own Country* and *The Tennis Partner*, two critically acclaimed books, is professor of medicine at Stanford. Born and raised in Ethiopia, his family originates from Kerala, India.

Walker, Alice (1944–), the eighth child of Georgia sharecroppers, received the Pulitzer Prize in 1983 for *The Color Purple*, the first African-American woman to win. In her book *The Same River Twice: Honoring the Difficult* she in part discusses her experience with Lyme disease.

Williams, Marie Sheppard was a social worker for 20 years and lives in Minnesota. *The Worldwide Church of the Handicapped* (Coffee House Press, 1996), from which comes *A Blight on Society*, was her first collection of short stories. All physicians should read this story, and this collection.

Zuger, Abigail writes for the *New York Times*. Born in New York City, she attended Harvard and Case Western Reserve, and trained in internal medicine at Bellevue. She is Associate Clinical Professor of Medicine at Einstein and an infectious disease expert. Her *Strong Shadows: Scenes from an Inner City AIDS Clinic* was published by WH Freeman in 1995.

Permissions

Every effort has been made by the authors, contributors, and editorial staff to contact holders of copyrights to obtain permission to reproduce copyrighted material. However, if any permissions have been inadvertently overlooked, the American College of Physicians will be pleased to make the necessary and reasonable arrangements at the first opportunity.

Bauby, Jean-Dominique: An excerpt from *The Diving Bell and the Butterfly*, translated by Jeremy Leggatt, translation copyright © 1997 by Alfred A. Knopf, a division of Random House, Inc. Used by permission of Alfred A. Knopf, a division of Random House, Inc.

Carver, Raymond: An excerpt from *Cathedral* © 1981, 1982, 1983 by Raymond Carver. Used by permission of Alfred A. Knopf, a division of Random House, Inc.

Gordon, Mary: An excerpt from *The Stories of Mary Gordon* © 2006 by Mary Gordon. Used by permission of Pantheon Books, a division of Random House, Inc.

Hemingway, Ernest: An excerpt from *The Short Stories of Ernest Hemingway* © 1925 by Charles Scribner's Sons. Copyright renewed 1953 by Ernest Hemingway. Reprinted with the permission of Scribner, an imprint of Simon & Schuster Adult Publishing Group.

Le Guin, Ursula: An excerpt from *The Wind's Twelve Quarters* © 1973, 2001 by Ursula K. Le Guin; first appeared in New Dimensions 3. Reprinted by permission of the author and the author's agency, the Virginia Kidd Agency, Inc.

About the Editors

Michael A. Lacombe, MD

Dr. Lacombe has practiced medicine for over thirty years in rural Maine and is former Director of Cardiology at Maine General Medical Center in Augusta. Editor of the "On Being a Doctor" and "Ad Libitum" sections of *Annals of Internal Medicine*, he has also edited the three volumes in the *On Being a Doctor* series published by ACP Press. He is the author of *Medicine Made Clear: House Calls from a Maine Country Doctor*, *The Pocket Doctor*, and *The Pocket Pediatrician*. A collection of his stories of medicine is forthcoming from the University of Maine Press. With Christine Laine, MD, he has edited the companion prose anthology to this volume, *In Whatever Houses We May Visit: An Anthology of Poems That Have Inspired Physicians*, published by ACP Press in 2008.

Christine Laine, MD, MPH

Dr. Laine is a clinician, researcher, and medical educator who has worked in medical journalism for more than a decade and is is Senior Deputy Editor of *Annals of Internal Medicine*. After receiving an undergraduate degree in writing, she completed medical school at State University of New York at Stony Brook, internal medicine residency training at New York Hospital Cornell University Medical College, fellowship training in general internal medicine and clinical epidemiology at Beth Israel Hospital Harvard Medical School, and a master's degree in public health at Harvard University. She co-edits the "On Being A Doctor" and "Ad Libitum" sections of *Annals* with Dr. Michael Lacombe. She is a Clinical Associate Professor of Medicine at Jefferson Medical College in Philadelphia, PA, where she practices and teaches internal medicine.